Medicine and Medical Policies in India

Medicine and Medical Policies in India

Social and Historical Perspectives

Poonam Bala

LEXINGTON BOOKS

A division of
ROWMAN & LITTLEFIELD PUBLISHERS, INC.
Lanham • Boulder • New York • Toronto • Plymouth, UK

LEXINGTON BOOKS

A division of Rowman & Littlefield Publishers, Inc.
A wholly owned subsidiary of The Rowman & Littlefield Publishing Group, Inc.
4501 Forbes Boulevard, Suite 200
Lanham, MD 20706

Estover Road
Plymouth PL6 7PY
United Kingdom

British Library Cataloguing in Publication Information Available

Library of Congress Cataloging-in-Publication Data

Bala, Poonam, 1958-
Medicine and medical policies in India : social and historical perspectives / Poonam Bala.
p. ; cm.
Includes bibliographical references and index.
ISBN-13: 978-0-7391-1322-6 (cloth : alk. paper)
ISBN-10: 0-7391-1322-4 (cloth : alk. paper)
1. Medicine—India—History. 2. Medical policy—India—History. 3. Social medicine—India—History. I. Title.
[DNLM: 1. History of Medicine—India. 2. Health Policy—history—India. 3. Medicine, Traditional—history—India. WZ 70 JI4 B171m 2007]
R605.B347 2007
362.10954—dc22 2007013071

Printed in the United States of America

™ The paper used in this publication meets the minimum requirements of American National Standard for Information Sciences—Permanence of Paper for Printed Library Materials, ANSI/NISO Z39.48–1992.

To

My father (late) Raghubir Narain

and my mother, Sharda,

for their support and inspiration in academic pursuits

Contents

Foreword

Medical practice and health policy are major determinants of well-being for communities and nations, and they are also barometers of social and political processes that reflect cultural values. The impact of religion, priorities of governance, access to medical treatment, and opportunities of various segments of society to learn and practice medicine define a broad set of interests related to policy, which suggest a framework for social analysis and study of the history of medicine. This book is concerned with such questions in developing a history of medicine on the Indian subcontinent over an immense span of time, concerned with the ancient period of *Vedic* and post-*Vedic* culture, Muslim rule, and British colonial rule.

Elaborating these interests in policy and social context also highlights the point that the quality of health in a population is determined by much more than medical theory or even medical practice. Consequently, a focus on policy to orient research on the cultural history of medicine is timely, as we recognize the value of thinking about medical systems in the broader policy contexts of health systems and social systems. A wide range of global issues suggest timely questions concerning health policy, development, and equity that have become prominent topics for rethinking India's health policy agenda over the past decade. During this period, questions about changes in Indian society and its health system have been motivated by many factors, such as changing expectations, the impact of public-private partnerships, reconsideration of resource allocation through changing health finance mechanisms, and increasing attention to the health of populations in an effort to recognize the broader interests of public health beyond treatment-oriented clinical practice.

The historical perspective over the vastly different periods considered by this volume aims to show how a cultural historical perspective enhances appreciation of the interactions between health policy and social contexts, and from that we also expect to be able to consider the relevance of implications in the present day. For example, with a controversy raging once again in Summer 2006 about reservation policies, merit, and equitable and effective policies for medical training, it is useful to consider the history of who could practice medicine, what kind of support they received, and society's views of these practitioners during the three epochs that Poonam Bala has considered. Furthermore, inasmuch as India is currently embarking on a major new task of developing capacities for public health training and practice, one expects that a historical account that places health policy in a social and historical perspective should help to explain what has been missing and what is needed to improve health systems.

Consideration of Vedic medicine identifies three types of medical practitioners, including surgeons (*shalya vaidya*), physicians (*bhishak*), and magical healers (*bhishak atharvan*), that is, three streams with a continuity that remains recognizable. The texts of *Ayurveda* indicate the responsibilities and a recommended approach for physicians' practice, and the *Dharmashastra* texts clarify the role of doctors in society from a more critical perspective. Subsequently, during the second period this work considers, Poonam Bala argues that *Ayurveda* received the patronage of both Hindu and Muslim rulers. Similar features of *Unani* and *Ayurveda* facilitated this cross-support of the two approaches. But that situation was markedly different from the competing interactions and antagonistic relationship that characterized this relationship of British colonial medicine and indigenous Indian medical traditions. As the colonial medicine predominated, sub-cultural hierarchies and differences enabled some segments of the Indian population to exert more influence through easier access into the Western-styled medical profession. The experience of several groups is particularly instructive, such as the *bhadralok* in Bengal and Parsis in Western India.

Scholarly study of historical sources through a modern lens that differs from the point of view that guided construction of the source materials makes for a very difficult task of analysis, even more so when considering the diverse epochs that concern this volume. Because the nature of available information is so different, the task remains a major challenge. The sources provide different kinds of information, which enriches historical study, but a strategy for synthesizing findings from these diverse sources is neither straightforward nor obvious. Nevertheless, expanding the scope of interests that guide research in the field to more carefully address the broader contexts of health defines a worthwhile goal and directions for historical research. Such scholarship is needed and needs to be encouraged.

Mitchell Weiss, MD, PhD
Professor & Head, Department of Public Health and Epidemiology
Swiss Tropical Institute, Basel, Switzerland

Acknowledgments

The period between the initiation of this project and its completion witnessed a proliferation of writings on various aspects of history of science and medicine, discussing the political hegemony, power and professionalization of medical systems in different parts of the world. The focus in most of these writings has been on alternative as well as biomedical systems, or Western medicine. In recent years, the professionalized biomedical health care system in the Western world has taken on new challenges of reassessing the growing popularity of traditional medical systems beyond the ethnic communities. *Ayurveda,* the Indian system of medicine, exists as a strong component of the emerging popularity of alternative" health care systems. Bearing this perspective in mind, this work provides a fresh look at the historical trends that may justify the broad clientele base, public support and acceptance in different regions around the globe, in addition to providing a comprehensive history of medicine and medical policies in India. Broadly, this is an attempt to unravel the trajectories of medicine in relation to the changing policy framework in Indian history. Essentially, it presents a comprehensive account of dynamism in medicine in one of the most ancient cultures of the world—a culture which exemplifies the coexistence of several medical traditions, or medical pluralism, guided by the pre-eminence various levels of training system and medical practitioners.

The work, although in development for several years, attained a final form during my tenure at Case Western Reserve University in Cleveland, Ohio, USA. Several friends and colleagues have helped me in the US and in India at various stages of this work. My special thanks to Kathryn Karipides, Associate Provost at Case Western Reserve University for going out of her way to simplify official formalities while I was in India, and to my colleague, Dr. Rhonda Williams for providing collegial support during the final stages of this work. Also, to my colleague, Professor Alan Rocke, for accommodating my periodic requests in the work place, and to Nancy and Marissa who have always been very understanding. I would also like to thank Angela Sloan and Brian Hanna, Library Assistants at the Kelvin Smith Library, at Case Western Reserve University, among other staff, for their help in procuring books at a short notice, when needed, and to the technical support from Rachel, Jared, and Aaron Shaffer at the Freedman Computer Center at Case Western Reserve University for resolving periodic, and sometimes severe, computer crises. To Chris at the archival collections in Allen Medical Library, at Case Western Reserve University, my thanks for allowing me access to rare books. The staff at the National Archives, Jawaharlal Nehru University, and National Medical Library, New Delhi, also deserve a special mention for their help.

I am deeply indebted to the Wellcome Trust, London, UK, for awarding me a research travel grant enabling me to collect important research data which otherwise would not have been possible. Thanks also to the Wellcome Trust Medical Photographic Library for allowing access to rare photographs in the section of History of Medicine. I am grateful to the staff at the British Library for their help in procuring rare documents during my stay in London.

I extend my deep appreciation to Jeff Brand, Manager, Corporate Communications, Pfizer Inc., New York, for allowing access to rare pictures, painted by the revered artist, Robert Thorn, and to Anna Gasner, Photo Archivist, Pfizer Inc., who tirelessly worked on reproducing these as immaculate images. To Uday Sahay, Director General, Ministry of Information, New Delhi, and Prashant Kaundiniya, I owe much gratitude for their timely help during the final stages of this work.

Last, but not the least, I reserve a special place for my mother, who has always been supportive of my academic endeavors, and for whom, appreciative words alone may not be enough. For any gaps in this work, however, I remain responsible.

Chapter 1

Introduction: Studying Medical Trajectories and Policies

> History of medicine was a facet of the history of mankind, linked with the history of the culture, art, creeds and philosophies, economy, technology, and sociology of each period, thus binding the physician's endeavor to man's yearnings, struggles, and conquests in each historical epoch.
>
> —Henry Sigerist

William Osler,[1] a noted physician of the nineteenth century, and the father of internal medicine, in his lecture,'Growth of Truth,' viewing science as inseparable from the discipline of medicine, observed a curious relation between 'history' and 'science' as follows:

> History is simply the biography of the mind of man; and our interest in history, and its educational value to us, is directly proportionate to the completeness of our study of the individuals through whom this mind has been manifested. To understand clearly our position in any science today, we must go back to its beginnings and trace its gradual development, following certain laws, difficult to interpret and often obscured in the brilliancy of achievements—laws which everywhere illustrate this biography, this human endeavor, working through the long ages; and particularly is this the case with that history of the organized experience of the race which we call science.

By this definition, all single events in science have led to the development of medicine. The development of scientific opinions in history, thus, should not be understated in this context. As Harvey remarked, 'opinion is the source of opinion.' Thus, Sir William Perkin and the chemists made Robert Koch's work possible which gave the science of medicine a new perspective for medical men of later generations; and Pasteur's achievements provided conditions that inspired Lister and his successful discoveries. The doctrine of specific diseases was seen as indispensable to a progressive image of the developing medical science. History of science is, thus, written more as the abstract force pictured as the ever triumphant conqueror of ignorance throughout the ages. In view of this, scientific development becomes a 'piecemeal process' through which individual scientific achievements are "added to the ever growing stockpile that constitutes scientific technique and knowledge. And history of science becomes the discipline that chronicles both successive increments and the obstacles that have inhibited their accumulation."[2] A critical assessment of the history of science, thus, entails a detailed study of man's scientific activities in relation to local society, social and political situation, and the ideologies governing these activities.

On a different note, history of science can also be viewed as "the history of the birth, life, and death of conceptual paradigms."[3] But what are these paradigms, and how can we place them in the context of history of science and medicine? Paradigms, explains Kuhn, are part of a conceptual system, sufficiently powerful to challenge and overthrow prior scientific thoughts as well as flexible enough to provide new problems to be resolved by the scientific community.[4] It follows then that the notion of the social nature of scientific thought, dictating that a new discovery can be and should be understood only within the background of the going paradigm and the difficulties that have arisen within it,[5] also calls for accepting the legitimacy of historical approach to the explanation of discovery. For an understanding of the growth of science in general, or medicine in particular, it is, therefore, imperative that we note the historical process which allowed the transition from the erstwhile supernatural basis of science and medicine and hence of the intellectual movements of Europe, to a more modern scientific approach to studying facts. These developments which took place in eighth- and ninth-century Europe changed the entire economic basis of society. Scientific achievements in the non-Western world, on the other hand, strengthened the scientific thinking as a result of their transfer to Europe. India and China offer good examples of these changes. Needham has a case in point when he describes how developments in China gave a new scientific world to Europe.

> In case after case, it can be shown with overwhelming probability that the fundamental discoveries and inventions made in China were transmitted to Europe, for example, magnetic science, equatorial celestial coordinates and the equatorial mounting of observational astronomical instruments, quantitative cartography, the technology of caste iron, essential components of the reciprocating steam-engine..., the mechanical clock, to say nothing of the gunpowder and all that followed there from. The overwhelmingly diverse discoveries and inventions had earth-shaking effects in Europe, but in China the social order of bureaucratic feudalism was very little disturbed by them.[6]

Accepting the veracity in the above definition, like most medical traditions of ancient civilizations, traditional Chinese medicine also is perceived in Western societies as "the continuation of an ancient, original an authentic tradition practiced widely as successfully over the centuries."[7]

Alongside changes in the scientific outlook, writings on the history of medicine also followed a significant trajectory in terms of the areas of research over a period of time. For instance, for a long time, historical narratives in the history of medicine focused on the 'history of great doctors and their marvels or discoveries.' In other words, great interest was shown in 'firsts,' or 'who discovered what first,' or the 'great discoveries and their discoverers.'[8] Earlier works on medical history were written by medical men themselves, thus providing a new foundation for writings in later years. Admittedly, the last decade has witnessed a gradual proliferation of studies on history of medicine, encompassing newer scopes of inquiry. Detailed as they are, these writings offer useful insights into history of specific diseases, of epidemics, of various aspects of health, medicine, and surgery, highlighting the transition to studying medical personnel and medical practitioners. In defining how these new areas of inquiry took their final form, I drew much inspiration from Porter and Bynum's[9] views on the relevance of social and cultural factors, and the role they played in modifying the medical profession in later years. Here is how they have summed up their opinion. "The once-common assumption of the essential benignity and triumphal progress of medicine has found its critics, resulting in greater concern to dispassionately scrutinize the social and cultural roles that the medical profession has played in the past."[10] Surely enough, medicine has been subject to severe criticisms; the growing interest in its history, testifies to this.

At this stage, it would be appropriate to provide some theoretical perspectives which characterize the emerging trends in studying medicine in its social environment. Until about a decade ago, understanding the concepts of health and illness in a social *milieu*, was visibly marginalized in the discipline of sociology of health and illness. Over the years, however, newer perspectives in social theory have renewed and altered the way in which issues of bodily experiences were analyzed in the humanities and social sciences. This book also uses an approach which cuts across three separate, yet interlinked, disciplines—sociology of health and illness, medical anthropology and history. Most recently, anthropology has provided new dimensions of studying disease and health by looking at ways in which "body symbolism is used in small-scale societies to integrate communities and define social relations and spatial relationships."[11] Lupton gives an impresssive description of how the three fields tend to blur in describing social phenomena including health and health care, medical encounter, capitalism and doctor-patient relationship, as some of the major issues. Reference is made to the influence of poststructuralism, feminist, and Foucauldian scholarship on constructing the human body through discourses and social practices in history that have allowed a closer alliance between sociology and health professions.[12] The popularity of the works of the French philosopher-historian, Michel Foucault, and the feminist scholarship on social construction of gender, and the political ideologies outlining gender roles in a medical context, propelled new interests in the body in historical, sociological and anthropological literary writings. Arnold's[13] pioneering work utilizes this approach to explain medical practices in relation to colonial power and hegemony in India. Generally speaking, studies on history of medicine in India have reflected a shift in the focus of historical inquiry from themes on public health and politics in British India

(Jeffery),[14] to a marked concern about British colonial power and hegemony through alteration of topography as a measure to vindicate colonial rule (Harrison),[15] or even regional studies depicting an interplay between medical knowledge and the empire.[16] Others have viewed the context of imperial decline as undermining contemporary notions of the degeneration of the colony.

The above studies, persuasive as they are in broadening our understanding of the imperial imperatives and their association with health and disease conditions generally, need to be revisited with a different outlook and portrayal of the role played by the political ideology in changing the character of the discipline of medicine in a non-colonial political environment. This study is written in the hope of bridging this 'literary gap' in identifying the government as the prime 'actor' in the dynamics of medicine during various historical periods in India. In view of this, India offers a unique example of an arena of interaction between the medical traditions and the ruling ideology—unique because not only it has had one of the oldest civilizations in the world, but also because it has been the home of several foreign rulers and invasions each of which was instrumental in shaping her institutions, traditions, and above all, her medical character over several successful centuries. Since with every new ruling and political ideology came the medicine of the new cultural group, a study of medical traditions in India represents an *acculturated* product of policies and plural medical systems. The study bears upon Kuhn's[17] approach to unravel the growth of medical traditions in Indian history, punctuated by changes in ruling ideologies which made transformations in scientific and medical paradigms a reality. It will be shown that with the advancement of the scientific era in historical studies, medicine seized the opportunity to re-establish itself under meticulous scrutiny by scholars with a new outlook in relation to humanity. Quite simply, how did the medical profession in India survive with the changing political odds? In trying to explain this argument, much of my work promises to discuss the dominant character of the political State in Indian history. In line with this premise, much of my work also promises to discuss the role of the political State in determining and shaping the character of medical science in Indian history.

In the literature of science, a general scorn for inventions and their inventors is not uncommon. The development of science, accompanied by medical science, as other sciences in the rest of the world, went through several barriers of acceptance and rejection by the ruling ideologies. By this definition, it is not surprising that in India, too, the growth of medicine and the rise of classical and scientific methodology in science were hampered by the orthodoxy. The development of the concept of the Earth as the centre of the universe illustrates our point. For instance, the heliocentric theory of the universe with the earth rotating on its axis daily and revolving around the sun once a year, was not accepted by scientists ad astronomers for several centuries. It was not until the early sixteenth century that Nicolaus Copernicus created a new trend and theory on the position of the earth in the universe. Copernicus postulated that "the sun is at the centre of the universe, and has three movements—a daily spin of its axis, and annual orbit round the sun, and a gyration on the earth's axis of spin to account for the precession of the equinoxes."[18] There were obvious links between medicine and religion which continued in later years of the eighteenth century. In addition, the ruling Church in the Middle Ages barred physicians from practicing medicine, quite like the *brahmanical* orthodoxy of ancient times in India.

An account of the history of medicine will be incomplete without allusion to the works of Sigerist, often described as 'a true artificer of history,' who propounded that

> the history of medicine must be first of all history, but always medicine as well.[19] It is a facet of the history of mankind, linked with the history of the culture, art, creeds and philosophies, economy, technology, and sociology of each period, thus binding the physician's endeavor to man's yearnings, struggles, and conquests in each historical epoch.[20]

Bynum[21] and Porter[22] have provided a detailed sketch of the development of the medical tradition in the Western world and changes with respect to State and society. Accepting this, the same analogy can be applied to India to gauge the trajectories of the traditional medical systems. Quite often, there have been claims of the Hindus in accounting for the historical antiquity of their medicine; records of the first system of medicine may be traced as far back as sixth century BC.

The relation between the *Vedas,* the earliest records of Hindu knowledge deciphering the life of early Indo-Europeans between seven and six millennium BC, and civilization was studied by nationalist and religious reformers, Bal Gangadhar Tilak, Surendranath Bannerjee in a similar manner as the ruins and monuments of ancient Babylonian and Assyrian historical past. The history of medicine in India, thus, takes us back to the cradle of civilization—the civilization of the Indo-European groups who made their way into India around the third millennium BC. Although, at one time, the claims of the Hindus to have the oldest civilization in the world, was dismissed by Western historians, the work of William Jones and Marquess Wellesley amongst others, provided a different perspective to Indian learning by linking it with the European past. These links were explained in terms of linguistic connections between Sanskrit, Greek and Latin, "a theory of the interconnection of ancestral languages, and of their monogenesis."[23]

Referring to the practice of medicine in earlier civilizations, Castiglioni[24] offers a lucid explanation in support of medicine in India which may be used to explain the trends in the evolution of medical practices. He remarks,

> India offers all the attraction of a large and marvelous museum in medicine as in other fields, the magic practices of the primitive people, the cult stones and trees, the belief in amulets and charms, the traveling physicians and ambulant doctors of Greek description, the scholastic, pedantic, dogmatic and the most modern type of specialists are all found in the actual active practice shoulder to shoulder. All the stages of evolution of science of medicine from instinctive, empirical,

> magical, priestly, religious, metaphysical and scientific practice, thus all the stages of evolution of medicine are represented in this country.

Given the antiquity and rich cultural heritage of medical traditions in India, tracing their trajectory, genesis, evolution and development as a professional body of knowledge seems like an arduous task. This entails, amongst other tasks, identifying a logical periodization of Indian history. For purposes of analysis, and based on available sources, I have chosen to study its evolution over three broad periods in Indian history each of which coincides with the change in the nature of the ruling State, the rise and fall of dynasties and of the instability of the political State. Although this is taken only as a working model, historians would doubt the validity of such a model, especially in the wake of current scholarly debates and post-colonial interpretations of Indian history. The first of these periods is the *Vedic* and post-*Vedic* period, which witnessed the development of medical verses and incantations as the healing base for various diseases. The post-*Vedic* period, as continuing from the *Vedic* period saw the proliferation of writings on medicine, and the codification of medical knowledge into *Ayurveda* (description follows later in chapter 2). The next phase in the development of Indian medicine was the period under the Muslim State, marked by an amalgamation or syncretism of *Ayurveda,* and *Unani* medicine introduced by the Muslim rulers. This was followed by imperial rule which is considered significant not only because it witnessed the inclusion of Western medicine in the therapeutic systems of India, but also because it saw a competition between various healing systems, hitherto unseen in previous periods. A brief note summing up the changing nature of the State and its impact on medicine will suffice at this point. The *Vedic* and post-*Vedic* periods impinge upon the development of the earliest writings, or the oldest repositories of Hindu culture, the *Vedas*; the post-*Vedic* period when the classical medical tradition was first codified by Indian sages and seers (600 BC), followed by the rise of Buddhism, Jainism and their struggle with the dominant *brahmanical* ideology to gain acceptance in society. Medicine was one part of the culture which, by its new outlook on man and nature, seemed to threaten the ruling orthodoxy. This explains why the ancient source books on Indian medicine that reach us today reveal a strange amalgam of science and religion. One can identify a rather lucid imposition of 'an assorted heap of religious and quasi-religious ideas and attitudes with no scientific significance whatsoever.'[25] The period also marked an interesting phase of struggle between medicine, its practitioners and the ruling ideology at a time when the newly formed State brought under its control various social and political institutions. The situation becomes clear as we move into the subsequent rule of the Muslims which witnessed the development of schools of medicine and chemistry in the neighboring Arab world, bearing a significant impact on the medical tradition in India. This was followed by more than two hundred years of colonial rule of the British, initially trading with India as the East India Company until 1857 when, after the Indian *Sepoy* Mutiny, the British took over from the Crown. The period assumed also significance from the point of view of the development of the scientific world in Europe which carved out phases of scientific development in India at the same time. It was in the seventeenth and eighteenth centuries that a systematic exploration of the world began to be put on a scientific basis. Moving to the late nineteenth-century British India, one notices a clear discontinuity from the previous periods; this difference is to be sought in the relative position of scientific developments and industry which made the period more interesting when Western and Indian forms of medicine for the first time were found in an ambiance of competition with each other. The period of 1750 and 1850 was one of progress for medicine not only in Britain but also throughout Europe which showed repeated calls for such a reform and professional uniformity.

The post-War period of the 1920s witnessed a new focus on the Indian outlook on the progress of science and medicine. 'Science,' generally, was seen as a universal framework which legitimized the colonial efforts, quite akin to Arnold's concept of medicine as a 'tool' of empire.[26] On another note, a recent work by Winther[27] argues that the use of opium as a medicinal product and as a necessity for trade in the late nineteenth century, reified issues of morality, culture and medical knowledge in a colonial setting. This also meant that the means of exerting power were also facilitated by popular acceptance of medical dictates of the colonial administrators. Admittedly, progress in science was a powerful ally to claims in colonial India.[28] For Indian nationalists in late colonial India, science

> was one ground on which a claim to abolishing the particular claims of 'nativeness' and consequent difference which was the basis of colonial constructions of its own superiority. At the same time, the scientist was an Indian scientist—the Indian part of it was relevant not in Indian science being separate from 'Western' science or science as a whole, but in that Indians could contribute as equals in the scientific world.[29]

Insofar as the profession of medicine, as a specialized occupation, is identified by its exclusive knowledge, skills, specialized and formal institutional training, special privileges, and position in the medical market place of consumers, its maintenance, continuity and improvement are part of a large formal political process. Elsewhere in the colonies of Africa, as much as in the Asian countries, politics and notions of racial comparisons influenced the thinking of medical authorities. Mental health was one area that was largely influenced by the way the colonizers viewed its causes and who it affected the most.[30] Notions of superiority of Western science could easily justify the racial basis of some diseases, such as malaria, typhoid and yellow fever.[31] However,

> when seen as part of a political process, however, knowledge and skill are claimed by a group to advance its interest. True or false the knowledge, disinterested or interested in the motive, claims of knowledge function as ideologies, and can be evaluated independently of their validity for their part in gaining public and legislative support for an organized occupation. Indeed, it seems likely that insofar as claims to knowledge and skill are essential elements in a political proc-

> ess which takes place in an arena of conflicting or competing claims from other interest groups, occupational or otherwise, it is highly unlikely that they can remain neutrally descriptive.[32]

In this study, I claim that as part of the medical professional traits, the existence of a willing clientele played a crucial role in determining the medical market in terms of popularity of medicine. Issues, however, become more interesting as we look into the nature of the clientele-base as medical practitioners, as lay-public and popular support, or even as nationalists who advocated their preference as a sequel to anti-imperial sentiments.

This work, it is hoped, will contribute to the recent emerging trends in interdisciplinary scholarship in the humanities and social sciences. As indicated above, it is a study of history of medicine that follows the flexible boundaries between anthropology, history and sociology. Some anthropological studies provide a cultural critique of the political and economic regimes in influencing health and medicine in different societies. Kleinman's pioneering work on Chinese culture and Taiwan explores the popularity of medicine as a business, simultaneously with the prosperity of traditional and folk healers.[33] The data in this study are drawn largely from archival primary and secondary sources. Given the nature of the study, they fall short of a subaltern perspective of reliance on oral tradition, considered indispensable to a post-colonial interpretation of Indian history. Where does the study of history of Indian medicine fit in relation to these new trajectories? In the absence of comprehensive and detailed literature on the status of Indian medicine during various phases in Indian history, a study such as this would provide a broad canvas from which the intricate nuances of medical developments can be traced and examined for more accuracy. A word on how dynamism in Indian medicine is perceived—a concept open to debates among scholars in various disciplines. Apparently, the near unanimous belief is that Indian medicine declined with the invasion of Muslims, and then later when the British introduced their system of medicine which seemed different from the extant medical systems. Although these reasons, initially, persuasive, left me with a doubt about what might have happened to medicine before the Muslim rulers went to India. The fact that this aspect has largely been ignored in historical scholarship, indicated the existence of eventful happenings in previous years. Earlier writings on history of medicine,[34] thus, opened up new avenues for research hitherto unknown before. They doubt the veracity of the argument that all was well with *Ayurveda* in the period prior to the advent of Muslim rule which falsifies the halcyon portrait of *Ayurveda* as portrayed in historical literature. What happened to medicine at the time? Did it degenerate, and if so, where did the decline begin? What were the sources of its decline? In answering these questions, a study of the nature and the role of the political State and its support or opposition to medical science in the *Vedic* and post-*Vedic* periods, becomes indispensable. This forms the theme of chapter 2 which is also devoted to examining State patronage in terms of famous practitioners patronized by the State, the famous medical texts written and if these were proscribed by the ideology, the nature of the State towards practitioners, and evidence of persecution by the State. Referring to State opposition to medical science, there is hardly any institution which does not meet with opposition in the initial stages of its development. In line with this trajectory, the fall in grace of Galileo's scientific credibility during the sixteenth and seventeeth centuries, and his condemnation in 1633 by the Church, suggests that philosophical and scientific discourses at the time were open to criticism by the Church and ruling ideology, although Paduan aristocracy tried to prevent his persecution at a later date. In this chapter, thus, my main concern is to see whether *Ayurveda* was really persecuted by the State, and to assess the veracity of the thesis that *Ayurveda* became comatose because of ideological and State intervention and opposition. In chapter 3, the issues are made more challenging with the arrival of the Muslim rulers and their system of medicine, *Unani*. Different as they seemed, initially, both *Ayurveda* and *Unani* shared a similar diagnostic and therapeutic framework for medical practice which facilitated an amicable co-existence. The history of Greco-Arab or *Unani* medicine in India is an area still under researched, although a recent study by Liebeskind[35] opens up new vistas on the conflicts between advocates of *Unani* medicine and Western or bio-medicine, arguing in defense of *Unani* as scientific and professional. The existing historical records that do exist are scattered in various medical works, and I hope I have done justice to the information by keeping analytical solecisms to the minimum.

Chapter 4 looks at the relationship between the colonial imperatives and indigenous medicine which at the time of British entry into India included significant aspects of theory and practice of *Ayurveda* as well as *Unani*. The added dimension in this chapter is the overlordship which was primarily hegemonic and colonial in nature, and which had produced an intellectual attitude as a result of scientific revolution in the seventeenth century, resulting in rapid strides in the field of science and medicine. An important feature of this discussion is the rise of intellectual consciousness amongst the clientele of medicine—a clientele which owes its origins to the preceding period of Muslims which facilitated its prosperity. In British India, the chief patrons of medicine, both indigenous and Western, were the local, urban elites represented by the *Parsis* and *Bhadralok*. At the height of the nationalist movement in India, the support base for medicine remained, but its leaders and practitioners developed a fresh outlook on medicine—'traditional' and 'modern' approaches marked the period so that by the end of the colonial rule, medical profession was seen as a combination of several medical systems or what Leslie[36] calls plural medical systems. Leslie's pioneering work on *Ayurveda*, challenged the near unanimous assumptions on indigenous medical traditions as closed and almost 'impervious' to progressive changes, thus enabling new inquiries into Indian medicine as professionalized, hence scientific. The existence of different levels of medical training and of medical practitioners provided several options within a plural medical setting, ranging from folk to popular, to learned secular and religious medicine.[37]

Science and medicine, which were once the privilege of educated urban elite, were now seen by the educated elites, and Indian nationalists as part of the cultural rejuvenation of India.[38] Claimed to be already scientific, it was declared that "only racial bias and a lack of objectivity prevented cosmopolitan medicine [biomedicine] learning from the Indian systems."[39] These claims also formed part of the emerging nationalistic interpretations of Indian history as a consequence of anti-colonial movement and nationalist struggle for independence. In the medical arena, the result seemed obvious: plural medical systems, several support groups, and a secure clientele-base which kept the practice of medicine in a perpetual state of dynamism, competition and accommodation in later years.

Chapter 2

Birth of Indian Medicine: State Support or Assault in Ancient Times?

> I have myself met with curious fragments of that primaeval work; and in the *Veda* itself, I found, with astonishment, an entire *Upanishad* on the internal parts of the human body, with an enumeration of the nerves, veins, and arteries; a description of the heart, spleen, and liver, and various disquisitions on the formation and growth of the foetus.
>
> —Sir William Jones[1]

The history of medicine in India begins with unraveling the pre-*Vedic* status of medicine, around the third millennium BC, followed by a *Vedic* period when the *Vedas*, the oldest repositories of Hindu knowledge, were written and compiled by sages and seers during the early stages of development of Indian society, and finally, the post-*Vedic* period when medical practice changed its approach and attitude to disease diagnosis and cure.

Indus Valley Civilization and *Vedic* Origins of Medicine

The most authentic evidence of the origin of Indian medicine comes from the excavations at the cities of *Harappa* (near Lahore) and *Mohenjo-Daro* (near modern Sukkur), and Lothal which together formed the Indus Valley civilization, the ruins of which were first unearthed in the 1920s.[2] The sites date from about the third millennium to second millennium BC, although the Bactrian document found in the northern region of Kashmir testifies to the existence of a mature civilization around the six millennium BC, incomparable to any civilization at the time. The sites reveal a socially, technically and medically advanced urban culture with well developed system of urban civilization, hygiene and drainage system extending along the Indus river (which now divides India and modern Pakistan). The town planning and architecture indicate a level of sanitation, hitherto unencountered in other ancient civilizations. Many streets and well-built houses with a systematic hygienic plan, and provided with an extraordinarily developed system of drainage have been excavated from the two sites. The near-perfect architecture indicates a high degree of consciousness about public health, and sanitation. The Great Bath at *Mohenjo-Daro*, for instance, suggests a penchant for purification through ritual rites which later occupied a significant position in orthodox Hinduism. The water in the Great Bath, perhaps, epitomizes the existence of hydrotherapy to 'preserve health,' quite akin to the Roman baths in later years.[3] Several therapeutic drugs of vegetable, animal and mineral origin for the cure of ailments (rheumatism) have been unearthed from the two sites. The discovery of cinnabar proves the claim of ancient Hindu sages as amongst the foremost scientists who knew the art of making mercury and its preparations. Other medicinal plants, which were later found in *Vedic* medicine, suggest that one may see the *Harappan* culture as holding the "seeds of traditional Indian pharmaceutical knowledge."[4]

Evidence suggests the usage of plants in various religious ceremonies, and the material artifacts also point to links with later medical knowledge. The seal of *Pasupati* (Lord of the animals) suggests the existence of *Rudra* as the divine physician, perhaps, earlier than the twin-*Asvins* (*Vedic* physicians).The downfall of this unique civilization came from about the middle to late second millennium BC (about 1700 BC), although reasons for its decay have been a subject of controversy, explaining environmental changes affecting natural water resources and flooding of Indus Valley as a major cause of this decline.[5] For some scholars, the invasion and eastward migrations of the Indo-European population around the second millennium BC completely decimated and abandoned the settlements, while others attribute the decline of economic prosperity as major factors affecting this once-flourishing great culture.[6] Thapar, an eminent Marxist historian, refutes any claims advocating the theory of invasion of northern part of India by another invading culture. She remarks that

> there is virtually no evidence of the invasion and the conquest of northwestern India by a dominant culture coming from across the border. Most sites register a gradual change of archaeological cultures. Where there is evidence of destruction and burning it could as easily have been a local activity and is not indicative of a large-scale invasion. The border lands of the northwest were in communication with Iran and Central Asia even before the *Harappa* culture with evidence of the passage of goods and ideas across the region. This situation continued into later times and if seen in this light when the intermittent arrival of groups of Indo-European speakers in the northwest, perhaps as pastoralists or farmers or itinerant traders, would pose little problem. It is equally possible that in some cases local languages became Indo-Europeanized through contact.[7]

History of medicine in India after that period then became a history of invasions by foreign rulers, each changing the character of medicine. Despite the controversial nature of debates on Aryan invasions, it may still be believed that they gave India the *Vedic* medicine, initially based on a lot of magical healing and later on a scientific method of investigation.

Vedas and *Vedic* Medicine

Just as the earliest visual evidence of an organized medical knowledge comes from the Indus Valley civilization, the earliest literary source of medicine in ancient times, likewise, is found in the oldest repositories of Hindu culture, the *Vedas,* which are also the earliest records of human civilization, and the sacred writings of the Hindus. The four *Vedas*, called *Rgveda, Samaveda, Yajurveda,* and *Atharvaveda* have hymns that show that *Vedic* Aryans migrated and settled as colonies in different parts of the world which later became centers of civilization in China, Persia, Egypt, Babylonia, Greece and Rome, and later in the south-eastern regions of Cambodia, Java, Sumatra. The sciences of Astronomy, Geometry and practical Anatomy were developed and cultivated more intensely by ancient Hindus as part of their daily life, largely influenced by religion.

Although primarily religious in nature, the *Vedas* represent the earliest period "in which a clearly discernible medical lore can be ascertained,"[8] written and compiled by sages and seers during the *Vedic* period which lasted from 2500 to 2000 BC. Apparently, the earliest evidence of medicine is found in the *Rgveda,* then later in the *Atharvaveda.* Because of their antiquity and the nature of the oral tradition contained in them, the *Vedic* texts have been most extensively researched for their philological contents. Even though they are not completely free of problems, they still provide a firm theoretical base upon which the history and evolution of the medical tradition in ancient earlier periods can be established. The *Rgveda* is almost primarily religious in nature, although it does contain hymns which eulogize the healing role of physicians—the twin *Asvins.* The existence of *Asvins,* however, does not justify the existence of a separate medical tradition in the *Vedic* period. In contrast, there have been assertions that *Vedic* medicine was 'archaic' and simple because the etiology of disease was ascribed to the supernatural. Concomitantly, healing practices consisted of imprecations against demons, enemies through elaborate rituals, charms, amulets, incantations for expelling diseases, sometimes 'necessitating spiritually potent and efficacious words, actions and devices.'[9] Sigerist, however, asserts that

> it would be a mistake to assume that Indian medicine in the *Vedic* period was only magical and religious. It had empirical and rational elements too. Even in the *Vedic samhitas*, the purely religious books, we find a reflection of anatomical, physiological and pathological views which are neither magical nor religious, and we hear of treatments which impress us as being rational.[10]

Accepting that rationality in medical practice existed in *Vedic* times, initial evidence can be seen in the writings in *Atharvaveda*, the oldest evidence of Indian medicine portraying more medical than religious content. It mentions hymns which allude to the predominance of charms, magical verses, and incantations for the cure of ailments. Besides, there are hymns which describe the use of catheters, and various skeletal parts of the human. Then there are hymns which carefully contain the procedures for application of drugs for the cure of specific ailments. The continuity in the medical tradition was because there was some similarity in the *Rgvedic* and *Atharvavedic* medical hymns contained in the two texts, since both conained a similar paradigm of therapeutic care. Thus, "an account of the *Vedic* gods, foremost among whom are twin *Asvins* playing the role of providing remedies, reflects the interest of the *Rgveda* in medicine."[11]

Early *Vedic* medicine was, essentially, based on a healing tradition of magico-religious beliefs and rituals, deifying demons that were believed to invade the human body, as a result of commitment of sin or breach of taboo. The role of the healer in the *Rgvedic* tradition then indicates that although the cure of disease was very much a 'case of the angry supernatural,' his knowledge of medicinal herbs cannot be discounted. For he was believed to be one "who repaired the fracture, suggesting that one of his professional activities was the setting of bones."[12]

Since the *Vedic* hymns were transmitted not by written lores but by memories and word of mouth, handed down to sages and seers over centuries, it has been a difficult task to ascertain their dates accurately. In some ways, they may be akin to the Iliad and Odyssey of ancient Greece, usually sung by bards before they were written down in a form that exists today.[13] Alongside social and economic prosperity, we also see a highly developed medical practice flourishing during the period. The hymns portray a well developed sketch of the migrating Aryans—their style of life and their interest in medicine. We hear of surgeons attending the battle camps and fields during the time of war between clans and tribes. We also hear of the existence of three groups of medical practitioners who, by virtue of their medical expertise and support, were able to flourish. The three groups consisted of surgeons (*shalya vaidyas)*, physicians (*bhisaks*), and magic doctors (*bhisak atharvans*).[14] Some major surgical feats seen in the removal of injured eyes, and replacing them by artificial ones, extracting arrow-shafts from the limbs of Aryan chiefs and soldiers, amputating injured legs and substituting iron ones,[15] show that medicine in ancient times was not a closed system or paradigm. What may be uncertain at this stage is whether medical knowledge had full fledged potentials of a medical profession the attributes of which become clear and focused as we move to Muslim and colonial periods.

Reverence for medicinal plants and nature was a marked feature of the healing tradition in *Vedic* period. Local flora was used in practices during a ritual performance, either as an agent to expel demonic attacks or as part of sacred utterances to give a healing touch. It is little surprising that *Rgveda* would list about one thousand names of medicinal plants, praising the uses of water in hydrotherapy. The rich armamentarium of indigenous plants formed the pharmacopeiac essentials of medicine in later years. Amongst the various surgical techniques employed by surgeons, an entire *Vedic* hymn is devoted to the treatment of phthisis, with descriptions of midwifery, child management and sanitation.[16] It is possible then that the beginnings of what later became 'rational medicine' were found in the *Vedic* tradition. Zysk claims that all medicinal plants were subject to investigation for their medical efficacy and their features were carefully noted which meant that medical thought was systematic in terms of categorizing diseases and in using empirical methods to cure them. It also meant a new direction in the medical outlook, or beginnings of an "empirical mode of thought, exemplified in their penchant for enumeration, so prevalent in later Indian philosophical, religious and scientific literature."[17]

Epics, post-*Vedic* Period, and Medical Knowledge

The end of the *Vedic* period marked the onset of the Epic period (2500 BC to 600 BC) or the golden age of literary and medical marvels, describing the events which led up to the composition of the two texts of Hindu religion—the *Ramayana* and *Mahabharata*. The two treatises, besides being religious texts, describe the extent to which surgery and medical practice had developed in ancient and post-Vedic times. The period, they mention, witnessed the prosperity of several renowned warriors, kings, poets and philosophers, and marked the zenith of Indo-Aryan culture. It was the period of *Ramayana* and "the rise of mighty kingdoms and empires, of extensive wars and conquests which culminated in the great war of *Mahabharata* when India shook with the armies of rival kings of *Pandavas* and *Kauravas* who employed infantry, cavalry, chariots, and elephants, and flying balls emitting the sound of a thunderbolt."[18] The two epics, which later became the basis of Hindu religion and mythology, confirm the existence of physicians attached to the royal courts, as well as army surgeons who were well equipped with the necessary medical and surgical instruments to look after the health of the troopers. Performing operations in the field was seen as a challenge to the medical expertise of army physicians and surgeons. Lord *Rama,* as mentioned in *Ramayana*, had a personal physician, a *vaid*,[19] and a surgeon, called *Sushena*, who took care of his health and medical needs. It also gives evidence of the use of *Sanjivani*, a medicinal herb used to restore consciousness from severe injuries in the battlefield. The epic *Mahabharata*[20] also confirms the existence of surgeons to take care of crisis situation, performing surgical operations in the battlefield, when needed. Advanced medical knowledge in terms of scientific principles of the circulation of blood also characterized the period.

We now know that the medical tradition in the *Vedic* period was not wholly magico-religious; it had empirical and rational elements too. The latter were given a new form around the sixth century BC when medical knowledge was codified into a new body of medical thinking, called *Ayurveda*. And since there were already elements of scientific thinking in *Atharvaveda*, codification also meant a transition from the *Vedic* magico-religious to rational therapeutics; *Ayurveda*, was defined as the science by the knowledge of which human life can be understood; *Ayu* meaning life, and *Veda* meaning knowledge. It is called *Ayurveda* because it demarcates the life-enhancing substances, qualities, and actions from those that are not.[21] Two most important sources that refer to the initial existence of the new medical tradition are *Rgveda* and *Atharvaveda* both of which indicate that *Ayurveda* was perhaps the oldest systematized form of medicine. By this definition, *Ayurveda* shares its antiquity with *Rgveda* and its secular character with *Atharvaveda*. But this might seem simpler than it actually was. The issue of possible links has raised several debates on whether *Ayurveda* was only an extension (*Upaveda*) of the *Vedic* literature or a separate system of medicine codified after centuries of scientific investigations. Despite these debates, the possible linkage is largely seen in terms of dealing with curing of disease and attainment of long life.

A clear relationship of *Ayurveda* to other *Vedas* is, however, yet to be deciphered since there are differing opinions on whether it would be appropriate to call it an *Upaveda*, or as an essential part of *Atharvaveda*. The fact remains that traces of organized medical knowledge are found in later *Vedic* literature, with undisputed origins in earlier *Vedic* period. By this measure, history of medicine in India is, a 'history of science of life,' or *Ayurveda*, and later systematized as the *Upaveda*. Despite its divine origins, *Ayurveda* reveals an awareness of scientific thinking and attitude of the early Indians towards life and health.[22]

The medical knowledge contained in *Ayurveda* is said to come from *Brahma*, the Creator and the fountain-head of all learning. The divine nature of the classical medical tradition is seen not only in terms of its revelation by Lord *Indra,* but also in its strength and further development by the divine intellect and vision of the seers. This is how medical knowledge expanded. New methods were continuously devised to consolidate and develop the traditional knowledge. Specifically, these included *Adhyayana* (study), *Adhyapana* (teaching) and *Tadvidya-sambhasa* (discussion with experts). It was imperative to study medical science by theoretical and practical proficiency. Teaching by oral didactic methods confirmed the knowledge of the teacher, and was essential for general growth of knowledge. It also ensured continuity from one generation to another, thereby maintaining continuity in dissemination of medical knowledge. The third method of discussion with experts created an atmosphere of dialogue and discussions with an exchange of ideas that helped to widen the basis of medical thought. *Caraka*, a revered physician practicing *Ayurveda*, has described in detail the method of *sambhasa* (seminar and symposia) which resulted in arriving at scientific conclusions; there is documentation of several seminars held on various themes in different parts of the country; discussions on the origin of man and disease afflictions were considered important for the purpose.

For Chattopadhyaya,[23] the origin of *Ayurveda* is not to be traced in the *Vedic* tradition, as Filliozat[24] would claim, but in the period following the *Vedas*, called the *Brahmana* or *Satpatha* period characterized by a systematic codification of medical knowledge. Since the *Brahmanas* were compiled at the same time, the philosophical basis of *Ayurveda* could not be left unchallenged by theoreticians of the former. Thus, according to the classical tradition, the science of medicine is not a "product of human thought but part of an eternal truth revealed by the gods to humanity, even though the divine character was not a regular feature of *Ayurveda*."[25] By this definition, it has no beginning in history and is complete from the start. Given the extent of medical knowledge contained in the *Ayurvedic* texts, the divine character of *Ayurveda* was perhaps, just one of the stages in the professional development of *Ayurveda,* and not an end in itself and in any case, its divine character did not hamper its popularity or even uninterrupted scientific investigations by medical authorities.

There are two versions of the origin of *Ayurveda*. According to one school, *Brahma* passed on the knowledge of medicine to god *Dakshapati* who revealed it to the twin physicians, *Asvins*, later to Lord *Indra,* and finally to *Bharadvaja,* a *Vedic* sage and composer of hymns. In the *Caraka Samhita*, he was selected by othe *rsis*, or sages, to learn the science of life from Lord *Indra*, and when he came back, other sages readily acquired the knowledge from him. *Atreya Punarvasu*, was one of his disciple sages who taught the knowledge of diseases and medication to a group of sages, one of whom, called *Atreya* instructed six of his students—*Bhela*, *Agnivesa*, *Jatukarna*, *Parasar*, *Harita* and *Ksharapani* to compile all knowledge on drugs and diseases in a complete treatise. Of these, *Agnivesa* became the foremost compiler of the codified system of *Ayurveda*. His treatise was later redacted by *Caraka*, and named *Caraka Samhita.*

The *Vedic* period of *Ayurveda* has significance when *Asvins* performed miraculous feats in surgery. This knowledge was passed on to Lord *Divodasa Dhanvantari*, the king of *Kasi*, through Lord *Indra*, and finally revealed to *Susruta*. Other sages who received this knowledge were *Aupadhenavqa*, *Vaitaqrqana*, *Aurabhra*, *Pauskalavata*, *Karavirya* and *Gopuraraksit. Dalhana*, the commentator, added to this list *Bhoja*, *Nimi*, *Kankayana*, *Gargya* and *Galava.* Each of these disciples composed their treatises but *Susruta's* excelled in its nature and content of medical knowledge. Further development in the science of *Ayurveda* was, thus, channelised through the two schools—School of Surgery (*Dhanvantari Sampradaya)* and the School of Medicine *(Atreya Sampradaya)*.

Vestiges of magico-religious therapy from the preceding *Vedic* medical tradition were seen to survive to a limited extent in the treatises of *Bhela*, *Caraka* and *Susruta.* In all these treatises, *mantras*, or religious charms with healing powers, have been used in the treatment of body sores and wounds, poison mental illnesses, fever, and in the preparation of medicinal consecrations. Given the limited use of these incantations, we are safe to assume that *Ayurveda* was essentially a separate medical tradition superceding *Vedic* medicine. For it also "provided rather more rational than magical and religious explanations of disease and cure. Although magical medicine did not completely vanish from traditional Indian medical lore, it was never to acquire the status in *Ayurvedic* treatises which it had enjoyed in the *Atharvaveda*."[26]

At this point, it is appropriate to relate the scientific development in *Ayurveda* to Kuhn's theory of scientific paradigms.[27] While studying this, we are faced with a conundrum. Can the divine character of classical *Ayurveda* be taken as a paradigm in itself? Perhaps, yes. After all, it was "a taken-for-granted conception of what the issue is, and how it is solvable."[28] By this definition, all medical issues were seen in terms of problems and their resolutions. The medical paradigm seemed irreplaceable and unchanging, until a change was demanded by newer methods of scientific inquiry. On the contrary, the absence of proper traits of progressive acquisition of new knowledge, and of new and better scientific alternatives, might otherwise not support any claims on the scientific nature of *Ayurveda.* It will be seen, in later chapters of this book that the scientific essentials of *Ayurveda* were highlighted when the latter had to prove itself and compete for professional monopoly in relation to Western medicine (alternatively, allopathy, 'occidental' medicine, or more lately, called bio-medicine). This will be discussed as we get to our discussion on medicine in colonial India. The sacredness of Indian medicine, once accepted, became an obstacle to fundamental innovations with regard to theory, particularly in ancient times when the religious orthodoxy proved stifling to the growth of medical knowledge; the truth is that despite a stumbling trajectory, *Ayurveda* was never completely a closed system of knowledge.

Popper vehemently maintains that scientific theories are the explanatory tools of describing the constitution of things in nature. For him "scientific enterprise is a persistent search for the truth about the constitution of things"[29] which means that "every assertion and scientific hyphothesis is merely a guess of conjecture."[30] If one were to accept Popper's view that science is characterized by its power to challenge and overthrow scientific conjectures in order to establish new ones, then the *Ayurvedic* medical tradition represented a scientific body of knowledge built up on continuous refutations of old theories, or a series of processes which led to its codification in the sixth century BC.

Ayurveda and the New Philosophies

The period of sixth century BC represents the classical age not just for Indian medicine but also for the rise of intellectualism and philosophical thoughts. The period was marked by the apparent shift in the practice of medicine from total reliance on scriptural and *Vedic* texts, to reliance on a new methodology based on direct observation of the patient's condition. This led to the founding of the *Atreya* School of Medicine and the *Dhanvantari* School of Surgery, and the subsequent rise of two classes of medical practitioners: one following the School of

Atreya, representing physicians, and the other following the school of *Dhanvantari*, representing surgeons.

The medical practice of *Ayurveda*, with its new outlook on diagnosis and therapeutics, came under the influence of different systems of philosophy that emerged around the sixth century BC; predominant amongst these were *Nyaya, Vaisesika* and *Samkhya*. Admitting that the bond between philosophy and science is the love of truth, artistic truth in the one case and exact correspondence to phenomena in the other, their relationship is best described in a disease situation, by Jones.[31] Jones provides an interesting analysis on the existence of what he calls 'enemies' of medicine. Like all true sciences, he says, medicine also has had in its history at least three enemies represented by superstition, pseudo-philosophy and rhetoric. The first two profess to solve mysteries; the third is an 'ornament' that often hides the truth instead of adorning it. This is how the three groups will handle a disease situation. The superstitious man might say, this is the work of a devil; the pseudo-philosopher will say, it is due to excess of cold, and the rhetorician will remark, disease is but a blessing in disguise. Contrary to this, a scientist will follow a different approach and will look for the *vera causa*, researching until he is successful in finding the cause and cure of the disease, or at least until he is satisfied with his scientific methods of combating the disease.

Some of the great Indian intellectuals developed their theories within philosophical paradigms which were concerned not with the affairs of the supernatural, but with an intellectual tradition of scientific analysis, largely ignored by Western scholars. The earliest system of philosophy that developed in India and had a major role in influencing the medical knowledge and practice of *Ayurveda*, was called *Samkhya* philosophy. The material cause of the world and the nature of the cause as determined by the effect, formed the basis of this system. The earliest accounts on this relationship is given by Jolly.[32] As an example, the theory of five elements in the universe—space, wind, fire, water, and earth as five elements of the universe also forms the basis of diagnosis and therapeutics in *Ayurveda* as *panca-bhuta* (*panca* means five, and *bhuta* means elements) constituting the material essence of the universe. The association of different philosophies with *Ayurveda* has been a subject of debate amongst scholars. At this point, an allusion to the debate between Chattopadhyaya[33] and Majumdar[34] on the philosophical aspects of *Ayurveda*, with attention to concepts of *karma* and transmigration of soul and how they altered the therapeutic essentials of the classical medical tradition, would be useful. Majumdar believes that the law of *karma* has been borrowed from *Nyaya* philosophy, while Chattopadhyaya makes two comments on the issue: first, the theory of transmigration of soul and *karma* evolved long before the emergence of emergence of *Nyaya* philosophy which, in turn, rejects any claim of *Ayurveda* borrowing the theory from *Nyaya* philosophy. Second, even if *Ayurveda* incorporates these concepts, the efficacy of therapeutics would be least affected by them. In other words, physicians in ancient period in India could prescribe effective palliatives for diseases which, otherwise, were incurable. This openly flouted the law of *karma* according to which an incurable disease is the result of bad deeds of previous birth.

The most apparent influence of philosophy on *Ayurveda* can also be gauged from a well known verse of *Susruta Samhita* which states that "in medicine, those with a broad view recognize the relevance of diverse points of view regarding the causes of what happens to human beings."[35]

Another system of philosophy which developed in opposition to the orthodox philosophies was called the *Lokayata* School with *Carvaka* as its founder. In literal terms, *Lokayata* means 'philosophy of the people.' The school, also called the materialist school of thought, with its focus on the identification of the soul and the body and the belief in the destruction of the former as a result of the destruction of the body, rejected the concept of reincarnation. Discredited by the exponents of *Vedas* and of Hinduism, their world view was atheistic and scientific, viewing mind as inseparable from the human body, expressing disbelief in sacrificial components of religious practices. With the denial of *karma,* thus, the school denied the existence of fate and the merits or demerits acquired in previous life. Since materialism was annihilated by Hinduism and the religious orthodoxy, the philosophical basis of the school did not develop further.[36] Followers of *Lokayata* denied the validity of any source of knowledge and believed in direct perception of facts and empirical data. For them, there was no God, no soul, and hence no reincarnation. It followed that *Lokayatas* denied all religious and moral values, free from any obscurity. Doubtless, they ridiculed the Brahmanical orthodoxy and its rituals as well as the authority of the basis of *Vedic* philosophy in terms of *sruti*[37] and *smriti.*[38] So what was it that led to a change in the philosophical thoughts of earlier men of science in India?

Absolute anarchy and the breakdown of ancient and traditional authority gave rise to *Lokayata*, or it may be that this was already a part of priest craft which found expression in the absence of traditional authority. Despite the diverging views on its existence, *Lokayata* characterized the epic period from sixth century BC to 200 AD, as an intellectual product of a long period of peaceful polity and authority. It resulted when control over people crumbled to an extent that "so many metaphysical fancies and futile speculations were put forward. We have the materialists with theoretical insistence on the world of sense, and the Buddhists with their valuable psychological teachings and high ethics."[39]

The *Lokayata* school, despite its material orientation which often posed a threat to the ruling ideals, is often regarded as the most influential system of philosophy, both in terms of a new outlook on life and in terms of influencing the practice of *Ayurvedic* medicine. The physicians, as a result of the new methodology of medical science, developed a materialist view of nature with emphasis on direct observation of facts and natural phenomena and the rational processing of empirical data. As keen observers of nature, *Lokayatas* were probably amongst the first to develop a framework for understanding the nature and medicinal value of various plants and herbs. Judging by this, it is plausible that Indian medicine gradually evolved from the early scientific knowledge and understanding of the *Lokayatas*. The vast pharmacopoeia and the pharmacological theory in *Ayurveda* is a sure marker of the scope of empiricism it allowed in Indian medicine.[40] Followers of *Lokayata* school observed a fundamental unity of man and nature, viewing man as a part of nature. Since man was believed to be of the same stuff of which everything in nature was made, nothing in nature was considered irrelevant for medical purposes. Admittedly, the theory occupied a central place in *Ayurveda*; the transition in the therapeutics remained a remarkable feature in the history of medicine. Since medical practice in *Ayurveda* was based on the utility of substances present in nature, it successfully developed new theories which would allow scientific investigations and empirical outlook, at the same time enriching the armamentarium of indigenous drugs. Known for their observational acumen, as seen in *prabhava*,[41] *Ayurvedic* physicians remained constrained in their freedom for medical practice. In an atmosphere of control by the State and religious orthodoxy, it is little surprising that the near 'stagnant' state of medical practice was nothing but a result of intervention of orthodox religion and the power of its followers.

A similar situation of control of medical knowledge, and a close relation between medicine and philosophy was seen in ancient Greece, especially in the fifth century BC; the forebearers of the latter were superstition and mythology although the theories and principles developed between 500 BC and 500 AD formed the basis of bio-medicine in later years. Similar to Indian medicine, the famous *Hippocratic Corpus*, a collection of over seventy works composed between 450 BC and 350 BC, contains a few chapters which show an obvious relation with superstition, and pseudo-philosophy. The latter includes those who abandoned superstition but adopted 'rational and unverified or unverifiable hypotheses.'[42] Some of these works also reflect the mentality of the scientific minds most active in that period. Between 600 and 300 BC, philosophy saw its birth in Thales, who saw all things as water, and maturity in Aristotle, although the credit of the notion of opposites and their blending to give rise to various disease situations in medical practice goes to *Alcmaeon* in his *Floruit*, composed around 500 BC; the latter, for the first time, describes the concept of health as follows:

> Health is a condition maintained by equality among the powers, the moist, the dry the cold, the hot, the bitter, the sweet and the rest, but an autocracy among these produces disease. For autocracy is destructive of one or other member of a pair. A disease occurs through excess of heat or cold (agent), because of too much or too little nourishment (cause or occasion), in the blood, the marrow or the brain (place). Sometimes, disease occurs in these from external causes, from waters of such and such kinds, or from similar cause. But health is a harmonious blending of the various qualities.[43]

While philosophy in the earlier times in India did much to alter the character of medical practice in the years following sixth century BC, in ancient Greece, the alliance between philosophy and medicine fell into a period of conflict towards the end of fifth century BC, achieving a rapprochement a hundred years later. This relationship is best noticed in three major works of the *Corpus—Nutriment, Regimen I* and *Breaths*, which provide a basis of health as resulting from proper adjustment of fire and water in human bodies.

It was because fifth–century philosophy had achieved success in certain spheres, dictated by its method and unchallenged system of its own, particularly in mathematics, that many enthusiasts were anxious to extend the range of its activity to include medicine alongside other natural sciences. This effort was, however, unsuccessful because the hypotheses of natural science are not to be apprehended intuitively, as are those of mathematics, but need to be led up to and worked upon by a gradual process that proved unfavorable to the Greek mind. In later years, however, more specifically between 400 BC and 300 BC, the influence of philosophy on medicine acquired a more acceptable character when metaphysics and physics gave place to ethics. New principles of conduct and moral etiquette took over from the unchallenged medical practice of yester-years. The first principles of conduct were formulated by Democritus, followed by Socrates and Pluto, and later by Aristotle for whom both metaphysics and natural science were significant features of any practice—either philosophy or medicine. Aristotle gave a new shape to ethics with a fully developed basis from where it descended instead of rising further until the great advances came up in the nineteenth century.[44] After Aristotle, the focus of philosophy shifted from all other branches of knowledge to the 'science of conduct,' based on the intellectual energy of the two great post-Aristotelian schools, the Stoics and the Epicureans. Both schools derived their physics from their ethics rather than vice-versa. It is possible that after Aristotle, physicians felt the need to develop a new line of thinking to handle the growing body of medical knowledge. So great was the emphasis on the way the physician conducted himself that his duty was defined not in terms of acquiring new knowledge of medicine, surgery and related medical areas, but in terms of his relation with his patients. Winning the confidence and esteem of his patients formed an essential feature of his medical practice. It was this confidence which finally gave way to the growth of scientific and medical knowledge. Nothing could be achieved without a proper ethical conduct. In other words, medical etiquette was considered far more important than any other form of etiquette; patient was more important than the medical profession. In the absence of an external force controlling professional conduct, medical etiquette in ancient times could easily be tarnished if the physician lacked a good relation with his patient. Personal honor for medical practice, thus, counted for more than the actual value for medical knowledge. Also, etiquette in Greek medical practice rarely, if ever, made literary publications of new discoveries as indispensable to medical practice, unlike in *Ayurveda* when success of medical knowledge was defined in terms of the medical compendia produced by the physician; individual discoveries were to be publicized to declare the success of the practicing physician.

The *Hippocratic Corpus* contains books, mostly anonymous needing a refinement in literary style. Almost all *Hippocratic* manuscripts reaffirm their focus on the significance of observation rather than on identifying the cause of the disease. The medical sects seem not to have been so sharply separated in thought as were those of philosophy, as seen in the work of the writer of *Anonymous Londinensis*, who divides medical theorists into two classes—one attributing diseases to residues which breed poison in the system, and the other attributing diseases to imbalance of body elements. The latter bears close resemblance to the class of physicians mentioned in the *Atharvaveda,* describing two types of healing art one of which attributed diseases to natural causes. Ancient medicine, was, thus, accepted as the greatest work of an unknown physician that validated the theory of body humors and their balance and imbalance as responsible for disease situations. Likewise, ancient physicians after 600 BC had much in common in terms of medical practice of Greek physicians with their insistence on accurate observation and scientific reasoning for medical judgments.

Ayurvedic Texts and the Classical Medical Tradition

The main texts of *Ayurveda* were originally written in Sanskrit, although English and European translations are now available, with translations into modern Indian languages. References to these have been made earlier, but what follows now is a detailed discussion on the nature of *Ayurvedic* texts. The earliest surviving textbooks include *Caraka Samhita*[45] (hereafter, *CS)*, *Susruta Samhita* (hereafter, *SS)*, and *Astanga Samgraha.* The former two are named after their founder, and the latter compiled by *Vagbhata*. The *CS*, the major compendium on the *Ayurvedic* theory and practice, was composed around 1000 BC, with different dates proposed for its composition. The final redactor of *CS* was *Caraka*, a physician at the University of *Taksasila*. *SS*, an *Ayurvedic* compendium on surgery was compiled by *Susruta,* a reputed *Ayurvedic* surgeon who existed around 600 BC as the 'Father of Surgery.' *SS* represents the epitome of ancient Indian surgery which expounds the concepts and skills in surgery prevalent at the time. The two medical compendia provide the basis for medical practice in Indian medicine, and "constitute the historically documented foundations of most *Ayurvedic* medicines."[46] *SS* reveals the extent to which knowledge of the application of drugs had advanced in ancient India. It also gives a detailed classification and nomenclature of diseases along with their etiology, diagnosis, and treatment; the treatise was translated into Arabic for a wider dissemination of medical knowledge outside India.

Although there were different schools of medicine in ancient times, they shared the same principle of causality of disease, the principle of natural rather than supernatural causation of diseases, and the principle of belief in curing the incurable diseases. The three principles were vital features of *Ayurveda*. In addition, the *materia medica* of *Ayurveda* represents a full utilization of environmental resources. The text gives an account of more than six hundred drugs for the cure of various ailments. One also finds a detailed description of medicinal prescriptions and therapeutic methods; the latter includes a description of various surgical processes for operations. Symptoms for a large number of pathological conditions have been discussed at length. *SS*, on the other hand, gives primary importance to surgery in medical science. Both *CS* and *SS* mention eight branches of medicine, which include therapeutics (etiology, diagnosis and treatment of diseases), surgery, treatment of diseases of the eye, nose, throat, ear, and tongue, infantile disorders, treatment of disorders resulting from administration of poisons, knowledge of mental diseases, knowledge of tonics and drugs, and knowledge of virilifics. Though indications of these are found in the *Vedas*, it is difficult to say when actually they were founded as definite specialties. Since these are described categorically in the *samhitas* of *Caraka* and *Susruta,* it is certain that the categorization took place right before the *samhitas* were given the present shape. In *Puranas*, the literary writings eulogizing the teachings of the *Vedas*, it is mentioned that divisions of *Ayurveda* took place in *Dvapara*.[47] The credit for this goes to *Dhanvantari*, although *Vayupurana* mentions that *Bharadvaja* is the founder of science and art of medicine which he organized into specialties and delivered to his disciples.

The manner of diagnosis according to *CS* was sound, and reflected a perceptive method of medical practice. It consisted of three steps starting from authoritative instruction by persons whose observations were not influenced by their personal likes and dislikes. This was followed by perception, which included observation by the physician himself followed by inference. The last step was based on the physician's experience of rational application of drugs. According to *CS*, a person possessing knowledge of the rational application of drugs was superior to the one with mere empirical knowledge of therapeutic substances. Besides, ancient physicians also could distinguish between curable and incurable diseases. The use of the opposites, that is, increasing what has diminished in the body, and diminishing what has become excessive, served as a basis for the application of drugs and prescription of diets, related to the belief that body disorders are caused by an imbalance in the substances present in the body.

The philosophical bases and their critical evaluation in relation to *CS* have been well propounded by Dasgupta[48] who views *Ayurveda* as a specific school of thought, interesting even to a student of pure philosophy. From his theory followed three groups, each viewing the relationship between *Ayurveda* and philosophy from a different perspective. These groups were represented by those who saw *Samkhya* topics in the contents of *CS*; [49] those mainly interested in the *Nyaya* theories expounded in *CS*; [50] and finally, there were those who remarked on the importance of *Vaisesika* doctrines in the *CS*.[51] An initial account of the philosophical basis of *CS* was also provided by Jolly[52] who deciphered the philosophical content of *CS* illustrating it with *Samkhya* doctrines. At the beginning of the twentieth century, historians of Indian philosophy were struck mainly by the *Nyaya-Vaisesika* influences, and viewed *CS* as the oldest text based on *Vaisesika* and *Nyaya* theories.

The complexity and advancement in medical practice is authenticated by eight special branches or *angas* of *Ayurveda* which include *Salya* (surgery or removal of foreign bodies including abnormal fetus, application of instruments, alkali, cauterization and diagnosis (and treatment) of surgical diseases, *Salakya* (deals with the diseases of supra-clavicular parts such as eye, ear, nose, mouth, *Kayachikitsa* (general medicine for treatment of patients afflicted with gods, demons with pacifying measures), *Kaumarabhrtya* (management of child, wet-nurse, purification of defective breast milk, and treatment of diseases caused by affected milk and seizures), *Agadatantra* (Toxicology and diagnosis and treatment of animal bites and other poisons), *Rasayanatantra* (prevention of ageing, promotion of life span, intellect and strength and alleviation of disorders), and *Vajikaranatantra* (removal of the defects of semen and sexual stimulation. Of these, *Kayachikitsa* dealt with principles of General Medicine, including in modern terms, pathology, diagnosis, therapeutic and dietetics. The tradition of *Kayachikitsa* occupied an important place in the School of Medicine led by *Punarvasu Atreya*, parallel to the School of Surgery founded by *Dhanvantari*.

As an important feature of surgical practices, *Susruta* recognized the imperative need of good knowledge of anatomy for the surgeon for which he recommended the dissection of human cadaver. The method he suggested for preparing the cadaver was complex, but indispensable at the time. It includes a carefully prescribed procedure :

> the dead body of a well built male adult, who has not died of a longstanding disease is to be selected, the intestine cleared of the faucal matter, then the entire body is wrapped with *Kusa* grass, fastened with rope, kept immersed in running water for seven days in a secluded place. Afterwards, it is taken out and using brushed made out of grass, hairs, reeds and bamboo spikes, the entire body scraped commencing with the skin, and observing all the tissues, thoroughly.[53]

Unrefined and rudimentary as this may appear to modern physicians, it indeed was a bold venture when touching a dead body invoked social boycott at a time when social control was equated in terms of Brahmanical satisfaction of medical practice. Thorwald marks this as "the oldest lesson in dissection known to History."[54] Gauging by the complexity in the type of surgical instruments used at the time, it is not surprising to note the successes which identified medical practice, made possible by the use of implements classified into—*yantras* (appliances, 104 in all) and *shastras* (instruments, 20 in all).[55]

In the Aftermath of New Methodology of Medicine: Encounters with Priestly Ideology

In discussing the influence of religious orthodoxy on the new methodology of medical science in ancient India, the work of Chattopadhyaya[56] cannot go amiss. Chattopadhayaya, in tracing the trajectories of development and decline of science in ancient India, believed that the ideological requirements of the society suppressed the latent potentials of Indian medicine as a science, and hence of its paradigm. Hostages were given to the counter-ideology, when the law-givers' demand for it became increasingly oppressive. These helped the scientists to evade, at least partially, censorship of the law-givers. But what happens to the theoretical positions once gained by science? These, Chattopadhyaya, convincingly demonstrates, are not entirely lost.[57] Instead, they survived in the intellectual atmosphere of the various philosophical thoughts, which dominated all spheres of knowledge.

We are now faced with a question. What is really meant by science in the ancient times in India? Gauging from the above discussion, the only discipline that promises to be fully secular with clear potentials of the modern understanding of natural science was medicine, which started off in *Vedic* times, and matured into a complete and codified body of knowledge in the sixth century BC. In spite of its humble beginnings, the nature of medicine changed from magico-religious therapeutics to rational therapeutics, or from *daiva-vyapasraya bhesaja* to *yukti-vyapasraya bhesaja*. As a result of the new outlook of physicians, in *Yajurveda*, the physicians come under strong condemnation, which continues throughout the later legal literature of *Apastamba* and *Gautama* belonging to a few centuries before the Christian era to the late commentators of *Manu*, including *Kulluka Bhatta*, of twelfth and thirteenth century AD.

It is significant to note that the mere knowledge of natural substances was not what *Ayurveda* regarded as important, but the adequate use of drugs or the rational application, called *yukti*, that was considered crucial; this was a key concept of Indian medicine. It follows that therapeutics in *Ayurveda* was based on the application of drugs, following a careful examination of the patient's condition. Empirical observation of the patient also included finding anomalies in medical theories and modifying them with better and more plausible alternatives. It was this challenging task of questioning medical knowledge for better application of its methods that threatened the religious ideology; the latter saw empiricism as a threat to priestly rules for practice, which accepted the existence of everything in nature as unquestionable, and hence not subject to scrutiny. At least, this is what seems to be the most likely explanation. Creativity of practicing physicians, thus, came to a state of comatose under the ruling priestly ideology. Since the earlier medical men viewed everything in terms of matter, they were placed near the *Lokayatas* who were regarded as heretics by the Indian law-givers, for they rejected the theory of *karma* and reincarnation. So deep-rooted was the animosity that the school declared the rituals of Brahmans a 'fraud,' and rejected the concept of supernaturalism. It declared that the endeavor to propitiate gods through religious ceremonies, as mentioned in the *Vedic* literature, is illusive. Subsequently, the physicians' rejection of scriptural declaration went against the religious beliefs of the priestly authorities. With the new focus on diagnosis and treatment, the physician began to rely more on the specific action of medicinal drugs to determine their effectiveness on the disease. By doing so, their implicit dismissal met with opposition from the ruling ideology. "The emphasis on supreme importance of knowledge based on direct observation was enough to annoy the spokesmen of orthodoxy, because it left hardly any scope for their advocacy for the implicit faith in the scriptures."[58]

At a time when doubts and scientific queries by the *Lokayatas* and Buddhists became severe, "when the authority of the sacred books was not merely tacitly set aside or undermined, but openly discarded or denied, and the institutions founded on them were abandoned and assailed,"[59] the orthodox piety enforced stringent and stifling measures to curb the materialist denigrations of religious order. And because medical science could not survive in this atmosphere, it was forced to produce medical literature with religious underlinings for acceptance by the ruling authorities. In addition to the supreme importance attached to the medicinal drug and its non-acceptance by Brahmans, the emphasis on dissection of corpse was also disfavored by the authorities. But without this, as *Susruta* claims, the knowledge of anatomy was incomplete and unsatisfactory as validated in his treatise, stating that "whoever wishes to practice surgery must prepare a corpse in the proper way and see by careful dissection every part of the body in order that he may have definite and doubtless knowledge."[60] Direct observation ensured the ultimate certainty of the knowledge of different organs of the body. The need to dissect the human body was facilitated by the rich empirical data collected and compiled for medical purposes—data regarding substances for treatment and on pathological symptoms. The rational application of drugs necessitated direct observation, the success of which was believed to depend on experience and dissection. Empirical observation (*prabhava*), as described by Meulenbeld,[61] thus, represented the observational acumen of *Ayurvedic* physicians. The correct action of therapeutic drugs was determined by four concepts which include taste (*rasa)*, post-digestive taste (*vipaka*), potency (*virya*), and specific action (*prabhava*). It was believed that through these four basic concepts followed by scientific inquiries and ways of resolving medical problems to empirical facts that the effect of drugs could be properly ascertained by the physician.

Assault on the new methodology of medical science with elements of rational observation continued until medical science was sought to be restricted to the base-born offsprings[62] in the hierarchical society. The art of rhinoplasty and bone setting, though reflecting the achievements of the time, suffered a decline as a consequence of the growing prejudice against dissection of human cadaver; stricture against direct knowledge was strongly annihilated by the religious orthodoxy in ancient times. Contact with dead bodies was tabooed by the lawgivers, and anyone who touched them was to submit to purification baths and religious ceremonies. Study of anatomy was, as a result, rendered very difficult, thus creating obstacles for the progress of medical science.

Continued hostility from the orthodox ideology and the various religious concessions offered by physicians in the medical literature written at the time, pose serious problems for historians of science in trying to understand the interaction between medicine and the State. No medical compilation was free from the influence of priestly domination which questioned their scientific purity. How did medical practitioners gain acceptance from the ruling State? The usual way of expressing their allegiance was to "submit to the priests and their scriptural role. Significantly, from this standpoint, the self-confident doctors compare themselves to the technicians—the cooks and potters."[63]

Here is how surgeons described in *SS*, in interpreting the success of medical treatment, would prove their subservience to the priests. "The physician, the patient, the medicine and the attendants (nurses) are the four essential factors of a course of medical treatment. In the absence of a qualified physician, the three remaining factors of treatment will prove abortive, like a religious sacrifice performed without the help of a Brahman."[64]

A similar relation between medicine and ideology can be observed in Greece, and other European countries where practice of dissection was relegated to barber-surgeons. In ancient Greece, disease was believed to be inflicted by god dictating that man's fate was entirely in the hands of the supernatural. This meant that physicians in the profession were not always successful in enriching or modifying their medical practice. In all likelihood, they were expected to attribute the divine cause, and hence a divine solution to the disease situation. Thus, "one must have recourse to a priest, divine, augur or other religious official, and restore health to the nation by the therapy of expiation. In such a causal chain, there is no place for a doctor working solely with non-religious means."[65] While medicine and medical practice in most ancient civilizations had achieved success to a large extent, they are believed to have grown in different social and political *milieu.* Taking Greek and Indian medical systems as examples, it is easy to decipher the main factor influencing their development. The practice of medicine in ancient Greece stressed the importance of theory, while Indian medicine believed more in the direct and empirical observation of medical phenomena.[66] The reason for ignoring the practical aspects of medicine was the general contempt for it by the new class that emerged in Greece around the fifth century BC, which meant that "the head was independent of the hands."[67] This also meant that theory bore no relation to practice for the leisured class. The job of collecting herbs for therapeutic purposes was relegated to manual workers or herb collectors ranking low in the hierarchical society. As a result, Greek physicians had limited experience in identifying useful drugs or their utility in therapeutics. In view of this, references to limited access to *materia medica* in the *Hippocratic Corpus* and the physicians' inability to expand the knowledge they possessed, remains questionable. The philosophical debates on various medical topics, however, indicated that the view of man as an epitome of nature was less significant in Greek medicine, which was indispensable for medical thoughts in Indian medicine. A firm knowledge of the nature and application of medicinal drugs was an essential prerequisite for a 'good' practicing physician. Elaborate descriptions of these can be found in most ancient texts, which made them more vulnerable for aspersions by the ruling State and law givers. The factors influencing the medical traditions in India and Greece appear to be the same—the attitude to manual work. In Egypt, the law-givers justified social and hierarchical norms by using social functions of superstition, and the idea of 'occult evil agency' in producing bodily disorders, as essential elements of social control.

The later *Vedic* literature—the *Yajurveda* and the *Brahmanas*—for the first time gives literary evidence of the hostility of the priests to scientific development. Of the two recensions of *Yajurveda*, the Black (*Krishna*) and White (*Sukla)*, the former is replete with detailed accounts of the denunciation of ancient physicians. *Taittriya Samhita*, a recension of Black *Yajurveda*, and *Satpatha Brahmana* also repeatedly mention the degradation of twin-physicians (*Asvins*) for their medical past, mingling with common people and for their commitment to people. The *Kathaka Samhita*, *Kapisthala-katha Samhita*, and *Maitrayani Samhita* (amongst other recensions of Black *Yajurveda*) declare *Asvins* as 'impure' because of their status as physicians and also because their profession entailed indiscriminate and unaristrocratic mixing with people.[68] This, however, did not rule out the possibility of differences amongst priests themselves, which became clear during the *Yajurvedic* tradition. Three schools of *Yajurvedic* priests existed then. *Caraka Sakha* School which produced the *Kathaka Samhita*, *Maitrayani Samhita* and *Kapisthala-katha Samhita*; *Taittriya* School which gave us the *Taittiriya Samhita*, and the School of White *Yajurveda*, represented by *Vajasaneyi Samhita*. The latter two clearly censured the writings of *Caraka Sakha* for their contents, although this may not have been based on the inclusion of *Asvins* and the pronouncement of impurity on them. The fact remains that *Asvins* were downgraded in the ancient tradition not because they were soma-drinkers, but perhaps, because the *Yajurvedic* priests felt threatened by the physician-gods and their high status in society. And in order to maintain their hierarchical position, several aspersions were cast against the *Asvins* which eventually proved inimical to medicine in its developing form.[69] But we also find that contact with dead bodies was tabooed by the law-givers in ancient India, and required elaborate religious ceremonies for purification.

Legal Wrath: Indian Medicine, Practitioners Estranged

Although difficult to ascertain in terms of the available sources, the legal contempt for *Ayurveda* and its practitioners can be traced as far back as the sixth century BC. If we were to go by the limited sources authenticating this development, it can be said that the law-codes of the earliest groups of Indian lawgivers represented by *Apastamba*, *Gautama* and *Vasistha* provided crucial evidence in this direction. Admittedly, the entire legal literature from the start of the Christian era to the period of *Manu* indicates a strong contempt for the emphasis laid on empirical knowledge in *Ayurveda*. And the usual way of expressing their hostility "was to declare the doctors as intrinsically impure human beings—so impure that their very presence pollutes a place, that food offered by them is too filthy to be accepted, and that even the food offered to them turns into something vile."[70]

The *Dharmasutras*, the law-codes of the earliest law-givers, were developed into *smritis*, oldest among which is that of *Manu*. *Manu's* attitude to physicians in ancient times reflects the prejudice against manual practice, and therefore, against craftsmen in general. Their very presence, according to *Manu*, was believed to destroy the sanctity of sacrifice for which reason surgeons were not allowed at sacrificial ceremonies. The legal contempt for *Ayurvedic* physicians seemed so intense that one is disturbed by the status accorded to the medical profession and its practitioners. Medicine, as a profession, was gradually regarded as too derogatory a profession to be followed by any member of a privileged class or the *dvijas*,[71] and was finally entrusted on a specific group of people born in violation of mating laws. The latter, according to the law codes of *Baudhayana*, were also called the *ambasthas*. Thus, notwithstanding its utility, the very basis and essence of medical practice was viewed as degrading. To add to the low status of physicians and surgeons, the law-codes also demanded penance of fasting as a result of offence if eating or even accepting food from a leather worker, carpenter, blacksmith, or a physician. Given the practical nature of medicine, ancient law-givers may not have refrained from recognizing the practical efficacy of medicine. However, the urestrained quest for knowledge and the questioning nature of medicine threatened the basis of the ruling ideology, and the usual way of controlling this was to declare the practice degrading.

Some scholars[72] believe that the legal attack on *Ayurveda* and its physicians cannot be justified by what is written in *Dharmasutras,* since the latter are not really law literature; their main purpose was to validate and preserve the hierarchical society by emphasizing in the texts the religious duties of man rather than legal aspects. Besides, the manuals were written by Brahmins, priests and scholars—the custodians of all literature—for the purpose of imparting instructions, and were not written as codes for practical use in the codes of law. In the law codes of *Baudhyana* and *Manu,* there is no mention of the *Atharvaveda*, the last of the four *Vedas*. Since the initial evidence of what later became rational medicine was found in the *Atharvaveda*, the law codes dismissed these as unimportant for the society. As a result, their discussions were limited to the three *Vedas*, with almost no association with rational therapeutics. But in spite of the weighty evidence adduced by several authors to show that *Ayurveda* was being downgraded by orthodoxy, we fail to find in the works of these authors any criticism against the *Ayurvedic* texts as such. Therefore, it can be surmised that it was not the craft of *Ayurveda* that the orthodoxy was against but that the latter were making sure that the *Ayurvedic* physicians did not claim a superior position in the social hierarchy. To this effect, beliefs on medical threat, pollution and purity were activated which, in turn, pushed status seeking *vaids* away from conducting renewed social investigations in medical science. Gradually, the *vaids,* became, purveyors of the healing art, much like the Hippocratic physician in ancient Greece.

The Emerging State: Where did Medical Knowledge Go from Here?

While the new form of medicine struggled to survive in an atmosphere of extreme hostility, the State and society in India underwent a series of changes which affected the trajectories of medical knowledge in later years. The changes occurred in two distinct phases. During the initial phase, the *Harappan* cities which emerged in the middle of the third millennium BC, declined some five to six hundred years later, only to re-emerge a thousand years later with new townships. Admittedly, very few elements of the old culture survived which means that the initial phase of urbanization had little connections with the new phase of development. The second phase of urbanization was goaded by the use of iron technology and its extension to the field of production, in a vastly different socio-economic *milieu.*

It was during the second phase when the migrating Aryan groups entered India, which coincided with the decline of the Indus Valley civilization. Indian society at that time was simple and comprised of warriors, priests and the common people. The first step in the direction of caste was taken when the incoming groups of people began to treat the *dasas*, or the original inhabitants, beyond the social pale. This led to the formation of a distinct hierarchical system, based on the four castes or *varnas*, with *Brahmans* at the top of the social ladder, followed by *Kshatriyas* (warriors), *Vaishyas* (merchants), and *Shudras* (untouchables) at the bottom rung of the social hierarchy, strengthened and perpetuated by virtue of birth in a particular social group. This was promoted by the transition from nomadic pastoralism to a more settled agrarian economy. Gradually, the increasing new settlements and the clearing of forests led to the emergence of a trading community aiding in the supply and exchange of goods which further enhanced the creation of powerful kingdom deriving revenue from agriculture. Here then was the rise of first cities in India. Childe[73] formulated the significant archaeological traits of what he termed 'Urban Revolution'—a term first coined by him in 1936. In 1950, he listed important archaeological traits accompanying the earliest city as follows:

> the first cities must have been more extensive and more densely populated than any other previous settlements,
>
> the non-food producing specialists were supported by the surplus concentrated in temples or royal granaries and were dependent on the temple or court. Amongst the specialists priests, civil and military leaders and officials absorbed a major share of the surplus and thus came to form the ruling class which conferred substantial benefits upon the subjects in the way of planning and organization.

The Emperor collected the surplus through various taxes imposed on the people. The later *Vedic* age witnessed the emergence of territorial monarchy concomitant with the transformation of the nature of kingship. The royal power increased, and now the king could even grant land with the consent of the clan. The king assisted by the Brahmans and the war-chiefs came to dominate the whole scene. The growth of cities led to further development of various forms of social and political institutions. The city then came to be seen as a community to which a craftsman could belong politically as well as economically. In order to maintain law and order and to maintain a formal system of social control, the ruling class was compelled to invent systems of recording exact and useful sciences, and once revenue administration was took shape, it necessitated the invention of writing and numeral notation. The new developments enhanced more authentic records of exact sciences including geometry, arithmetic and astronomy.

With the expansion of city life, political power also grew. But it was very much aligned towards the temporal power because people were loyal in maintaining the social order. In this case, the social order was dictated by the State. The production of surplus, which is a necessary prelude to the change from village to city, divided people into various social classes. It was in the sixth century BC that contradictions began to develop between the settled tribal organisations (constituting the republican areas) and the new political phenomenon, the monarchy. The period also witnessed an increasing growth of towns, an impetus to which was given by the increasing trade, facilitated by the introduction of monetary system between India and the neighboring countries; the founders of the two great religions—Buddhism and Jainism—belonged to one of these republics as a result of which the two gained considerable support in the republican areas. Since the monarchs followed the Brahmanical theories, they were reviled in rural areas with active supporters of Buddhism. This may have led to the increasing disputes between the monarchs and the followers of its rival faith. For Buddha, the most effective way of achieving salvation was in small monastic groups which would allow for instruction of moral precepts. The establishment of mendicant orders, however, posed a threat to the Brahmanical order of religious specialists. At this time, Buddha and his followers declared the Brahmanical practices and sacrificial rituals as 'violent' and inhuman, at the same time questioning their special and natural authority to read the *Vedic* texts.[74] Between 600 and 300 BC, the intellectual climate of India was also characterized by the rise of various schools of metaphysics and of the ascetic sects.

The period also marked the beginning of the mercantile system in India. The emerging town and urban culture was marked by an exponential growth of scientific knowledge. The period was also marked by the infusion of spirit of rationalism in all spheres of knowledge. In any case, the city was not considered fit by Brahmanical custodians of knowledge or for any higher and spiritual thinking.[75] Literature written at that time, thus, tended to be the work of professional urban littérateur who invariably 'belonged to the leisure class.'[76] However, literature remained a 'close preserve of the class in power,' and private literature was not accessible to the common man, a proposition typical of all creative Sanskrit literature so that its patronage could be conveniently summed up as a method of conspicuous consumption. Included in this development was the science of geometry which had religious origins developing from sacerdotal exigencies. The science of construction of altars, called *Sulba*, emerged from the necessity of having altars in specific size and shapes during *Vedic* sacrifices. It may seem apparent that *Vedic* sacrifices were dictated by priests and hence, were offered complete patronage. This meant that the science of geometry developed gradually over a period of time with the increasing interest in *Vedic* sacrifices and support from the priests which required an advanced knowledge of developing altars. Mathematics, on the contrary, had no religious affiliations. This was because Indian scientists had already devised the mathematical implication of zero. The earliest surviving mathematical texts are *Baksali* Manuscript, whose author remains unknown, and the *Aryabhatiya* of *Aryabhata*, composed around 400 AD.[77]

Reflecting on the art and practice of medicine in the ancient times, one comes across several instances of hostile encounters between the Brahmanical ideology and the *Ayurvedic* physicians, and the usual manner of evading hostility to gain social and ideological acceptance was to give concessions to the ruling ideology. Thus, most medical compilations written at the time had religious underlinings to placate the priestly thinking.

The literary writings of *Dharmasutras* and *Dharmasastras* not only disfavored medical practice for its rational approach, but also depicted a rural bias in their literary writings, and for the same reason, *Baudhayana* declared that the city was not deemed suitable for spiritual and moral growth; cities do not create a congenial environment for any kind of spiritual gain. Thus, while on the one hand, medical knowledge was gaining a momentum and inspiration for new knowledge and medical practice, the expansion of city life hampered its growth. In more general terms, towns and cities were quite closely associated with oppressive officials. The traditional Brahmanical attitude of 'rural bias and urban antipathy' was, perhaps, more assertive in that the basis of social and economic life remained largely agricultural; *Ayurvedic* physicians were only one part of ideological expressions of antipathy.

Buddhist Ideology: A New *Home* for Medical Science

With its more humanitarian ideology, Buddhism, by this time, had gained popular appeal amongst the oppressed social groups in rural areas. The other side of this appeal was that Buddhism became unpopular when it questioned the *Brahmanical* ideology and its authority over the *Vedas*. Its advocates challenged the validity of the lawgivers (*smriti* writers) and the priestly authorities. As an attempt to purify the ritualistic mandates of *Ayurveda* formulated by its physicians to gain acceptance by the Brahmanical ideology, Buddhists formally adopted *Ayurveda* as a therapeutic form of medicine. The espousal of *Ayurveda* and the expansion of Buddhism then became closely intertwined during the reign of Buddha (563–483 BC) with repeated efforts to purify, restructure and reform the ancient and rich cultural medical heritage of India.

Of all the occupations during the period of Buddha, thus, the profession of medicine appeared to have been honored the most. One finds a frequent appreciative mention of the activities of Jivaka, a royal and personal physician to Buddha, and son of king Bimbisara of Magadha (in the north-eastern part of India). *Jivaka* was a reputed physician at the University of Taxila, or Taksasila, (now in modern day Pakistan), the major seat of learning during Buddha's time. He was known for his expertise in sub-specialties and surgical techniques, especially cranial surgery for which he was often provided a high honorarium. He was considered the most skilled physician of his time, and stories about his achievements earned a reputation in Buddhist territories of Magadha in northeast India, Benares, and Peshawar near the Khyber pass (between modern day Pakistan and Afghanistan) in northern Asia and China. Buddha's interest in medicine formed part of his compassion for living beings and for the sick, also reflected in the various texts comprising the *Vinaya pitaka*, a collection of rules for Buddhist order. He declared that "Whoever, O monks, would nurse me, he should nurse the sick."[78] *Mahavagga*, a Buddhist text provides an invaluable source for the history of Indian medicine; it contains a comprehensive section on medicaments indicating the highly advanced level of knowledge of *Ayurvedic* physicians of the time. Also the medical care described in the *Mahavagga*, as Chattopadhyaya says, appears to be reminiscent of the system of rational therapeutics of the *CS* according to which, of the four factors, on which the success of medical treatment depends, one is the patient himself. It was the last factor which aroused a reaction from the priests against the basis of medical practice, hence justifying their continued contempt for medical practice. Moreover, the omission of the law of *karma* from the text as a justification for curing the incurable diseases, was sufficient to annoy the Indian orthodoxy because it formed the basis of all religious and priestly literature. As a reaction to this, Taxila, renowned for its excellence in the cultivation of medical science, was considered an impure place of learning by the ruling ideology. In contrast, one also comes across a physician called *Akasgotta Vejja*, who did well under Buddha, despite expressions of hostility. Another physician, *Nagasena*, figures in the *Milindapanhal*, a Buddhist text composed during the first century AD.

Notwithstanding the way Indian medicine and its practitioners were eulogized by advocates of Buddhism, the Buddhist period may not have been completely unaware of the supernatural undertones hitherto encountered in the early *Vedic* period. The following passage published in the Academy[79] indicates these obvious linkages:

> The 'rain-charm', translated by Prof. Buhler, is certainly Buddhistic, but appears to conform, for the most part, to the North Buddhist type. The mantra, or charm, contains a list of words which the translator thinks are the names of various plants to be used as ingredients for an oblation; but the Buddhists did not offer any sacrifices and oblations. These terms, therefore, may be merely magical or talismanic words, such as we often find in North-buddhist sutras, and are probably epithets of Siva's counterpart Durga. In the usual invocations, we find these magical terms in the vocative case.[80]

In the post–*Vedic* period, we find several changes in the political climate of the country. Buddhism gradually established itself in India, thus intensifying the hostility of Brahmans to Buddhist patrons. The rise and spread of Buddhism meant the decline of Brahmanical dominance. Brahmanical ideology, it is said, never accepted the growth of Buddhist faith, although at a later date it was counted as one of the *avataras.*[81]

Buddhism flourished well under the *Mauryan* kings and about the first or second century BC, followers of Buddhism actively sought support from royalty and the wealthy urban merchant class. *Mahayana* Buddhism was recognized as a religion which gradually spread to the adjacent regions too. Ashoka, a Hindu emperor of northern India (third century BC), and a benevolent monarch, impressed with Buddhist ideals of moral and ethical behavior, ardently supported the growth of Buddhist religion, around the third century BC. He built temples for *Siva* and monasteries for Buddhist monks. Under his rule, both Brahmanism (*Saivism*) and Buddhism flourished and co-existed, and even claimed the same persons as their devotees. He established several charitable institutions for the care of the infirm. Since Ashoka embraced Buddhist ideals of compassion for all living beings, he founded hospitals for animals too, and sent out missionaries to propagate the ideals of Buddhism. The spread of different branches of *Ayurveda* to neighboring and foreign regions was, thus, facilitated through Buddhist monks. Ninivaggi mentions that "there are extant documents cut in rock that display Ashoka's edicts directing embassies to be erected in foreign lands and ordering Buddhist missionaries to travel within and outside India to disseminate the teachings."[82]

Ashoka's edicts speak of his view on *dharma*, or social and moral obligations of man, based on tolerance and non-violence, which meant that the practice of animal sacrifice in rituals was disfavored by his followers. As a result of shared ideals, there were visible signs of the beginnings of a rapprochement between Brahmanism and Buddhism, as well as the popularity of *Ayurveda* with the spread of Buddhism outside India.[83] The initial enmity between the two religions emerged out of different interests in the two faiths; while Buddhism catered to the ethical needs of the human being, offering no provisions for rites and rituals, Brahmanism catered to the religious needs. Buddhism demanded from its followers a commitment to amity and moral life with faith in Buddha as the liberator of mankind from the worldly sorrows. As a result of these ideals, study of anatomy and dissection of corpse was strongly discouraged by Buddha and his followers, although hospitals and educational institutions were established for medical studies.

Buddhist interest in medicine found expression in the establishment of a university in Nalanda, in the city of Patna in the northwest region of Bihar, where medicine was introduced as separate area of study, alongside literature, law, commerce and other areas of humanities. There are records which illustrate that Chinese travelers to India often spoke about the rich and diverse cultures in India, with about 10,000 students and 1,500 teachers at the University. The later Buddhist period witnessed the development of the science of alchemy and metallurgy. Described as the rational age of India, the period was known for tremendous intellectual activity in arts and literature, as well as in scientific technology. Medical science, too, flourished well during this period.

The accidental discovery of the *Bower* Manuscript in 1890, named after its discoverer, Lieutenant H. Bower, was a landmark in the history of ancient medicine during the time of Buddha, in terms of the medical knowledge prevalent at the time. The Manuscript is claimed to be written by writers of Indian origin, most probably Buddhist monks traveling to different parts of the world for missionary and other philanthropic purposes. Despite a perceived irregularity in the contents, it contains an impressive description of internal medicine, of patients, diseases and administration of medicine, of cures for eye, throat along with a manual for prescriptions.[84] The subsequent period, the reign of the *Sungas*, witnessed a revival of Brahmanism as a result of an anti-Buddhist spirit of the ruling ideology. By the time the Greek rulers came to India, which was shortly after the downfall of *Sunga* dynasty, Buddhism had obtained a strong hold and was even welcomed by the existing foreign rulers. Some of the Greek rulers, it is believed, professed great faith in Indian medicine, especially for diseases that Greek physicians were unable to cure. Alexander, who had gathered eminent physicians in his army pavilion, depended upon Indian physicians, especially for treatment of snake-bite amongst his Greek soldiers. Impressed by their medical skills, Alexander returned to Greece with a few *Ayurvedic* medical practitioners.[85] Following the Greeks and *Sakas*, both of whom patronized Buddhism, the *Kushanas* were staunch supporters of Buddhism. They spent lavishly on the erection of stupas, temples and images of Buddha in several parts of India. *Kanishka,* an emperor of *Kushan* dynasty, also embraced Hinduism. The age of *Kushanas*, thus, was regarded as a period of great missionary and literary activities. *Nagarjuna*, a great exponent of *Mahayana* doctrine, and *Caraka* existed during this period; the latter in Chinese sources appears as the court physician to king Kanishka, around 100 AD. He was a renowned alchemist and a successful physician, and is often associated with the redaction of *SS*. Kanishka had his kingdom close to Taxila in Peshawar, and was an ardent supporter of *Mahayana* Buddhism, dictating self-development through social compassion. He encouraged the translation of *Ayurvedic* works into Chinese which made easier the entry of *Ayurveda* into China (Luoyang region) through Buddhist monks traveling into India. By the end of second century AD, royal interest in propagation of religion and medicine led to the establishment of Buddhist monasteries outside India simultaneously with the popularity of Indian medicine.[86]

A significant achievement of Indian medical practitioners at this time was marked by the inclusion of metals in the *Ayurvedic* pharmacopoeia, initiated by *Nagarjuna*, an alchemist, priest and a philosopher of eighth century AD, known for his excellence in the science of the preparation of medicinal mineral substances, as the Father of iatrochemistry. How did *Nagarjuna* achieve fame? How did *Ayurveda*, as a body of knowledge, benefit from his works? Up to this time, most medical interventions of *Caraka* tradition were derived from an herbal or plant-based pharmacopoeia, while physician-surgeons of the *Susruta* school excelled in various surgical approaches. *Nagarjuna* directed his efforts towards expanding the therapeutic armamentarium by constructing a mineral-based repertoire of active, healing substances. Many heretofore toxic substances, like mercury, were processed in complex ways using the innovative techniques of the *Nagarjuna* school, to render them nontoxic and suitable for human consumption. This paved the way for a new range of therapeutic interventions which characterize modern practice of *Ayurveda* in India. The brilliance of *Nagarjuna's* contributions, however, extended far beyond this and encompassed a qualitative advance in Buddhist theory and practice with an especially productive literature, in medicine, philosophy and religion.[87] Most certainly, Buddhist ideology viewed physicians and surgeons with great esteem as though liberating them from previous experiences of non-acceptability and ideological hostility. With the popularity of *Ayurveda* and princely efforts in improving its essentials, it should be little surprising that the Brahamanical hostility of yesteryears toward Buddhism intensified at the time.[88]

During the reign of the Guptas, worship of images of Buddha with elaborate ritualism became a universal practice and a notable feature of the Buddhists during the period. The period was also marked by the growth of Brahmanical cults like those of the *Bhagvatas* and the *Saivas*, alongside establishment of several monasteries. The *Gupta* emperors patronized Brahmanism, yet showed a marked tolerance towards Buddhism. This fact of common patronage to the two faiths, was largely responsible for initiating a rapprochement between Brahmanism and Buddhism.

The rulers' interest in medicine also found expression in the increasing number of compilations written and redacted during the period. Important *Ayurvedic* texts, *CS* and *SS* were redacted in this period. A noteworthy achievement in the field of medicine during the reign of Guptas was the compilation and renovation of earlier texts, albeit with limited knowledge of new practices; most of them were based on the physicians' rich data on herbs and their uses.

Vagbhata, a physician existing between the fifth and sixth century AD, summarized *Caraka's* work into eight chapters; his work later came to be called *Astanga Samgraha* or *Astanga Ayurveda.* We also know of a physician called *Dhanvantari* who existed at the courts of king Vikramaditya, receiving full patronage of the State. Support to the two faiths continued in the subsequent dynasties of Hindu rulers. Harshvardhana, a liberal patron arts and sciences, helped bring encomiums to philosophers, sages and of advocates of Buddhism and Hinduism.

Gupta and post-Gupta periods are known for their continued support to compilation and redaction work by earlier men of science. Evidently, these were not free from Brahmanical bias, as reflected in a later redaction of *SS* which mentions the subservient status of the doctor in relation to the priest. Also, the manner in which *SS* explains the relation between the doctor, patient, medicine and nurse—the four factors on which depends the success of medical care—is a sure marker of the manner in which ancient physicians made concessions for the priests to gain social acceptance. The text says that the three factors of treatment would be ineffective in the absence of a physician, like a religious ceremony performed in the absence of a priest. Another instance of religious concession is apparent from the extant *CS* which omits the inclusion of *Bharadvaja* for his belief in the laws of nature as opposed to the unchallenged laws of the *Vedic* scriptures. The later redactor of the text dropped *Bharadvaja* and began anew with *Atreya*, and in order "to add apparent conviction to its loyalty to the norm of orthodox piety, special chapters were added to the text for loudly proclaiming the theory of soul and its salvation."[89] One cannot but accept the continued dominance of the Brahmanical ideology during that period. Since the period also saw the acceptance of the hierarchical society in India, it strengthened the Brahmanical hold over Indian society, with new measures of granting land to Brahmans. Medical science and practitioners continued their work of compiling and redacting medical texts in trying to find a niche in the social order.

Around the eighth or seventh century AD, the growth and popularity of *Mahayanism* led to an increasing emphasis on prayers, incantations and rituals. It incorporated many folk beliefs, and "in doing so, the Buddhists made a clear approach to Hinduism,"[90] to such an extent that the distinction between the two became tenuous. The introduction of *tantrism* in Buddhism as the new form of religious practices and incantations further narrowed down this distinction, but the re-strengthening the hierarchical bse of society showed signs of a declining influence on Buddhism.

Fate of Medical Practice: Preliminary Reflections

Accepting that medical science in ancient times declined as a result of the superimposition of religion and superstition on science, what proved more fatal for Indian medicine was the offering of ransoms by its practitioners to the counter-ideology so as to prove innocuous in the eyes of the Indian orthodoxy and to make their compilations acceptable to them. The growth of hierachical interests of the ruling orthodoxy, set a greater challenge for medical science in proving its 'loyalty' to these aspirations; this is evident in the literary writings of the time. The *brahmanization* of medical science affirmed the orthodox orientation of secular medical knowledge. The transmission of medical knowledge from the deity to humans via a pantheon of Hindu gods and semi-divine and human individuals legitimized the control of knowledge by the ruling State. And because medicine was the first science that opened itself up to a material outlook of man and nature, alongwith its handmaiden materialist school of *Lokayata*, it became the first 'casualty' of religious hostility. This was believed to be the most serious internal cause of near-complete decadence of Indian medicine. Nevertheless, there were serious attempts at disguising a mythological veneer to medical practice, when the opportunity arose. The practicing *vaids* in Hindu courts, some of whom were known *Ayurvedic* exponents, justify our claims of the existence of secular medical practice outside the realm of religious orthodoxy. Common support to Hinduism and Buddhism added to the apathy towards medical men. The beginnings of a rapprochement between the two faiths can be traced to the Mauryan dynasty of which we know that the rulers actively supported the establishment of Buddhist monasteries along with Hindu temples. Besides, the reign of the Guptas also brought about the re-establishment of Hinduism as a distinct religion. It is agreed that with varying degrees of concession to religious orthodoxy, the paradigm of *Ayurvedic* medicine remained unchanged. During the Buddhist period, anatomy and surgery receded into the background, but the study of medicine, chemistry, metallurgy flourished well not only as distinct disciplines, but as an integral part of the philanthropic avocation of Buddhist philosophy and ideology. The practice of medicine and the humoral theory were left unaltered, though practice of dissection fell into the background. Moreover, the compilation work in the Gupta and post-Gupta periods did not result in noticeable scientific breaks, since the scientific paradigm remains unaltered, and as such no significant addition characterized the medical compendia of the period. Although medicine was most certainly a '*brahmanic*' science in its initial years, practising *vaids* who listened closely to the objectives of the orthodoxy, distanced themselves from polluting agents, or how else could they have been so enthusiastically patronized by several royal Hindu courts. The fact, however, remains that the *Ayurvedic* texts remained, in the pharmacopoeiac essentials, unaltered with the passage of time from the days they were originally conceived.[91] The use of the religious metaphor here or the dropping of a non-religious preceptor there did not alter substantially the contents of the codified texts of *Ayurveda,* although it did limit incorporation of medical ideas into the intellectual tradition without a veneer of Brahmanical mythology. Judging by these criteria, it might be logical to surmise that by modern science standards, though *Ayurveda* was patronized by the State, it did not gain pre-eminence in terms of scientific and medical progress, the hallmark of modern medicine, nor was there any noticeable regeneration of its scientific essentials.[92] Can we then say that State patronage does not necessarily rejuvenate a science? Can we then also say that the State often patronizes an art after it has been estranged by science, especially if it does not threaten the basis of the State? Alternatively, it is possible to surmise that indicators of assessing levels of medical progress were written differently at the time. Answers to these questions will be taken up in the following chapters of the book.

Chapter 3

Expanding Medical Practice: Patronage Systems under Muslim Rule

> By the grace of God, I have established one hospital where rich and poor are treated alike. For diagnosis, treatment as well as diet and medicine, learned *hakims* are always present. The expenses for food, medicine, etc., are met from the royal purse, by a grant by the king himself; and to the patients whether they are local residents of the town or strangers, upper class or lower class, free treatment is given.
>
> —Firoz Tughlaq (Tibb-e-Firuz Shahi)

On the status of science and technology during the Muslim rule in India, George Sarton, a pioneer in the history of European science, viewed Indian science as "stifling of Hindu culture and patronage of learned men of Arabic and Persian sources by Muslim emperors."[1] Rahman,[2] however, negates this view on the basis of the social, cultural and ethical factors which were an integral part of Asian scientific and technological thinking. He falsifies studies on the history of science and technology in India which portray a distorted view with a 'European-centric' vision. Early writings on this period were influenced by what was happening in Europe at the time, and since the medieval period in Europe was also viewed as a period of much decadence of knowledge, major scientific developments in any part of the world were largely seen as obscurantist, mystical, spiritual and, hence, devoid of any rational or scientific elements. It is little surprising then that developments in India also were rendered inconsequential in the scientific world.

Here is how we see the transfer of knowledge between eminent scholars in India and its neighboring regions at the time. During the tenth and eleventh centuries, there was rich cultural exchange between Arabic, Persian and Sanskrit scholars which facilitated the development of knowledge not only in areas of astronomical and mathematical sciences, but also in medicine. *Al-Biruni's* works present fine examples of some of the preeminent scientific works. The following discussion will unravel the processes and systems of support which paved the way for scholarly, medical, and literary achievements at the behest of Muslim royalty.

Royalty in Succession: Policies and Medical Science

The Muslim rule in India is often associated with noticeable changes it seen in the traditions, customs and religious faiths of India. The initial interest of Muslim rulers in India was primarily political and trade, both of which found expression with the arrival of Arab traders on the south-west coast of India, the Malabar Coast around the seventh century AD. Some scholars attribute the development of Hindu religious thought to this association during the period.[3] The impact of Muslim rule at this stage, although initially slight, assumed enormous proportions with the rule of Muslim Turks in the twelfth century which broke the long established reign of Hindu rulers. Their scepter was, however, taken over by the Afghan rulers who built and expanded their empire close to the middle of the fifteenth century. After a long lapse, sometime by the sixteenth century, the "élan of Muslim proselytism had died away; the tendency was now, apart from moments of passion of fanaticism, to live and let live. The Turkish enthusiasm for conquest and empire-building had wilted under the hammer blows of Taimur."[4]

It was at this stage of total confusion, conflict and loss of interest in expanding the imperial administration that the first *Mughal* or Turkish chief, Babur, went to India in 1517, with the successive rule continuing well into the beginning of the eighteenth century. The Muslim kingdom provided several opportunities facilitating the prosperity of Indian medical science in its art and practice. It was in this period that faced with new challenges of a new medical system, *Ayurveda* could easily identify parallels in diagnosis and therapeutics of other medical systems. Needless to say, the period also represented the most propitious time for *Ayurveda*, for it received maximum fillip for research and medical writings, not only by the ruling ideology, but also equally supportive *Ayurvedic* and *Unani*[5] practitioners and socially successful groups in the form of middle classes as patrons of medical practice. The set of processes became apparent under the aegis of the Muslim rulers from the eleventh to eighteenth centuries.

It is known that prior to the introduction of *Unani-Tibb*[6] medicine into India, there was a fair degree of exchange of *Ayurveda* and the Arabic world. Greek physicians had a strong influence on Arab medical thought. The Persian physician, Avicenna (980–1037 AD), for instance, compiled the works of Hippocrates and Galen into what eventually became the Canon of Medicine, and later the pre-eminent medical text for both the Muslim world and the entire Latin West until the seventeenth century.[7] His main work based on the theory of medicine is called, *al-Qanun*. Avicenna's contemporary, Razes was a prominent figure in the history of medieval medicine, known to be bold enough to "refuse to surrender to the authority of Galen's erroneous doctrines."[8]

As the most prolific writer, Razes is recognized by his *al-Hawi*, a manuscript which appeared after his death in 923 AD, and till date is identified as the most important and comprehensive Arabic compendium on medicine. After the fall of Greece and Rome, the Greek manuscripts were either lost or destroyed. The works of Hippocrates and Galen, however, were transferred to Constantinople from where the knowledge preserved in these manuscripts gradually spread to Arabia and the erstwhile Persia (now Iran). In Persia, the new form of medicine contained elements of both Greek and Indian medicine, further encouraged by the Nestorians.[9] After repeated Islamic conquests, medical knowledge finally went into the hands of Arabian authorities during fifth and sixth centuries AD. The body of knowledge that took its final form under the Arabic influence was named *Unani* medicine, variously called as Ionian Greek by its Muslim advocates (signifying its origin), and Greco-Arab by European scholars. The earliest Arabic medical writer was Ali Rabban, known for his *Firdausul-Hikmat* (Paradise of Wisdom)—a book providing a comprehensive summary of *Caraka Samhita, Susruta Samhita, Nidana Samhita and Astangahrdaya* written in 850 AD. This is how scholars perceive the syncretic accommodation of Arabic and Hindu medical ideas which formed the bulk of medical knowledge in *Unani* medicine. "Arabic tradition was a continuation and revivification not only of Greek science, but also of Iranian and Hindu ideas."[10] With these virtues, it is hardly surprising that Hippocrates, in his *Materia Medica*, recommended indigenous plants of medicinal value for use in the cure of various ailments which also figured in Sanskrit works.[11] Prominent amongst these were *Sesamum indicum (tila), Nardostachys jatamansi (jatamansi), and Boswellia thurifera (kunduru)*. The virtues of Indian medical knowledge were also recognized by Galen, whose scientific works and discoveries paved the way for modern medicine, and by Aetius, a reputed physician from Mesopotamia whose works on diseases of women derived largely from Indian drugs. Galen published his work on the dual qualities of all foods in the form of 'hot' and 'cold' foods, which were borrowed from India. Browne[12] sums up the relation in greater details as follows:

> Arabian medicine is that body of scientific or medical doctrine which is enshrined in books written in the Arabic languages, but which is for the most part Greek in its origin, though with Indian, Persian, and Syrian accretions. Its importance lies not in its originality, but in the fact that in the long interval which separated the decay of the Greek learning from the renaissance, it represented the most faithful tradition of ancient wisdom and was during the dark ages the principal source from which Europe derived such philosophical and scientific ideas as it possessed.

A series of invasions and subsequent destruction of flourishing Persian and central Asian cities under the Mongol rulers, Chengez Khan and Timur, led to a mass exodus of scholars and physicians into their neighboring countries. India at the time was projected as a neighboring region and in close proximity was seen as a country with a rich intellectual history of previous Hindu and Buddhist rulers. It looked more accommodating and congenial for scholars from Persia. It is a truism that *Ayurvedic* physicians, by the time the Muslim rulers went to India, had gained enough support through the existing clientele, providing them ample opportunities to utilize Indian drugs in their practice. This also supports Ninivaggi's claim that "these reputed *Ayurvedic* physicians were invited to Jundishpur and Baghdad to teach and organize hospitals."[13]

Several *vaids* treated intractable diseases which had baffled the medical knowledge and skill of their foreign counterparts. The influence of *Ayurvedic* knowledge on Arab and Greek physicians was so extensive that the writings of Avicenna and Razes were translated into Latin in thirteenth century AD for use as textbooks in various institutions in Europe. So also the works of Hippocrates and Galen were translated into Arabic. Baghdad, in particular, was the centre of intellectual and scientific activities under the aegis of Harun-Al-Rashid, a keen patron of medical science.

The period of Muslim rule was, thus, made more interesting by the arrival of *Unani* medicine and the establishment of Muslim rule in India. The co-existence of *Ayurveda* and its 'alien' counterpart (alien in its origin) provides a broader perspective for an understanding of the potentialities of dynamism in *Ayurveda*, for it led to extensive contact and interaction between two different, yet similar, medical traditions. Since the two were coexistent, a study of medicine in this period of Indian history would throw light on the nature of policies and attitude of the rulers towards *Ayurveda*.

Unani and *Ayurveda*: Literary Marvels under Royal Patronage

Although, under Muslim rule, a strong emphasis was laid on the propagation of *Unani*, it will be useful to take a fresh look at *Unani* medicine in the light of its support systems and State patronage, and its interaction with *Ayurveda* in order to get a larger understanding of the potentialities and dynamism of ancient medicine. For we know that by the time *Unani* medicine went to India, it represented an interesting gambit of an 'eclectic' medical system; 'eclectic' because it represented the best elements of Persia, India, China and other regions of central and southern Asia, taken from the Greeks by the Arabs who modified and enriched it on the basis on their observations and experience. The system was later organized on sound lines by the Mughals.[14]

The decline of the Greco-Roman Empire did not end the spur in scientific activities, kept alive Muslim rulers in previous years. Annshirwan (530–579 AD), for instance, established a medical school with a hospital at Jundishpur, exemplary of exchange between Indian and Greco-Arabic forms of medicine; medicine here was practiced on the basis of *Ayurveda*. Caliphs, as patrons of literary tradition, were also advocates of Hindu learning. Works of *Caraka* and

Susruta, including significant ones in gynecology, gained prominence through translations in Arabic made possible at the behest of the Caliph.[15]

The first Muslim rulers went to India in 711 AD; thereafter, the influx and exchange of *Unani* physicians continued for several centuries, culminating in the Mughal empire the rulers of which were ardent supporters and patrons of all medical activities. Medical practice and practitioners, thus, reached their pinnacle of performance under the aegis of the Muslim rulers, even though it meant identifying and promoting therapeutic drugs for specific ailments. Providing incentives and conferring honors to physicians were symbolic of royal appreciation of medical activities. This also attracted reputed *vaids* and *hakims* from different parts of India and neighboring lands. The rulers often conferred upon then high salaries, to encourage them to improve the healing art. Delhi, the centre of activity of the Sultanate rule, also became a center of 'culture and glory surpassing even that of Baghdad.'[16] Allauddin Khilji (1296–1321 AD) had several eminent *Unani* physicians in his courts. Successive rulers also had Muslim and Indian physicians who took active part in contributing to the development of *Unani* literature. A large part of this literature consisted of translations and summaries of important works, including those of *Ayurveda*.[17] The major achievements of *Ayurvedic* and *Unani* physicians were quite enthusiastically listed in the medical manuscripts produced under the aegis of Muslim royalty. In a congenial work environment such as this, *Ayurvedic* practitioners were satisfied by the encomiums achieved through State recognition of medical practice. It may appear at the outset, that the Muslim royalty recognized its physicians, *hakims*, brought from Persia and other regions, and encouraged them to develop literature on *Unani* medicine by consulting media sources. In later years, however, efforts were made to look into the significant marvels of *Ayurveda* by contact with Indian specialists in *Ayurveda*. It was as though the successive rulers realized the value of ancient medicine and allowed their *hakims* to translate the Indian medical texts into Persian.[18] The first such translation was called *Tibbe Firoz Shahi*, compiled during the reign of Firoz Tughlaq. *Hakims,* we know found employment at the royal courts; we also know that *Ayurvedic* physicians worked in the hospitals with practicing *hakims*. Both classes of physicians worked together in the medical institutions and clinics founded by the Muslim emperors, which suggests that although *Ayurveda* went through phases of restricted growth in previous years, almost reaching a state of comatose in an orthodox environment, its scientific essentials were recognized by the royalty, even if it meant perpetuating their personal interest. This enhanced the quality and extent of support medicine received, thus enabling the two medical traditions to flourish and co-exist. However, it was during Akbar's reign that the two traditions received the greatest fillip.[19] Scholars believe that during the early period of Muslim rule, Indian medicine languished for want of State support,[20] and continued so until the accession of Firoz Tughlaq to the throne in the fourteenth century. This was probably best seen in terms of the support and sponsorship for producing a Sanskrit work on astronomy, *Yantraraja*, by Mahendra Suri.[21] From the reign of Firoz Tughlaq onwards, several literary writings on *Ayurveda* were compiled and translated.

The earliest written documentation of *Unani* physicians and their achievements at the Muslim courts comes to us through the work of Ziya-ul-Din-Barani, a historian at the court of Firoz Tughlaq, in his *'An Account of the Physicians of Alai Period.'* The treatise mentions the existence of Maulana Badr-ul-Din Dimishqi, who taught the art and practice of medicine to *Unani* physicians in the city of Delhi. Similarly, the *al-Qanun* and *Qanuncha* of Maulana Hamid Motraz exemplify the eloquence of the medical knowledge of *hakims*. In addition, Mahachandra Tabib abd Jaja, an eminent Hindu physician practiced medicine with an unmatched accuracy, unparalleled anywhere in India.

The reign of Altamish (1212–1236 AD) attracted several *Unani* physicians from the neighboring regions into India. With aspirations of establishing a successful medical practice, some of these physicians set up their own clinics where they got popular support, while others took pride and were fortunate to offer their services to the kings and princes at the royal courts. Henceforth, Delhi, as the capital of the *Sultanate* Dynasty, became an important centre for intellectual activities. The economic prosperity and political stability during the Khilji dynasty under the rule of Ala al-Din Khilji (1295–1315 AD) opened up favorable opportunities for a successful medical practice in India. The subsequent rule of Mohammad bin Tughlaq (1325–1352 AD) witnessed an increasing number of compilations by *hakims*. Mohammad Tughlaq, often described as a great scholar, a lover of literature, and a dabbler of science, supported the publication of *Majauai-i-Ziae* by one of his courtiers, Ziya Muhammad Mubarak. The treatise provides a detailed account of the knowledge and practice of medicine in that period followed by a description of the humors and anatomy of the human body. It also includes chapters on different diseases and surgical procedures, has 221 folios, and draws largely on the works of Avicenna, Galen and *Ayurveda,*[22] thus recognizing the value of ancient medicine; a separate chapter was added later to incorporate the essentials of medicine advocated by *Nagarjuna*. Muhammad Tughlaq's rule is also identified by the establishment of clinics and hospitals for the poor and infirm; at least eighty hospitals and about twelve hundred physicians are listed as State employees.[23]

Firoz Tuglaq (1351–1388 AD), like his immediate predecessor, had a thorough knowledge of *Unani* medicine, was a good bone-setter and compiled a medical collyrium, *Kuhl-e-Firuz-Shahi,* enlisting the drugs for the cure of eye ailments. He extensively patronized *Unani* medicine by establishing and reorganizing clinical institutions hitherto left by his predecessors. He also encouraged the publication of *Tibb-e-Firuz Shahi*, and attended to patients in a hospital founded by him in Delhi, called *Dar al-Shifa*. The hospital cost him about 3.6 million *takas*. Monetary support to new hospitals was a salient feature of Firoz Shah's rule.[24] Food, medicines, and other expenses were paid by the villages especially cultivated and endowed for the purpose. Available evidence records the foundation of thirty medical schools and about a hundred hospitals throughout the country under his reign. The following passage[25] from his biography indicates the extent to which the royal State valued medical art and practice:

> By the grace of God, I have established one hospital where rich and poor are treated alike. For diagnosis, treatment as well as diet and medicine, learned *hakims* are always present. The expenses for food, medicine, etc., are met from the royal purse, by a grant by the king himself; and to the patients whether they are local residents of the town or strangers, upper class or lower class, free treatment is given.

Medical compositions under Firoz Tughlaq's reign provide ample evidence of his deep fascination for medical art. Prominent amongst these texts are *Shifa al-Khani*, *Tibb-i Shahabi*, *Rahat-al-insan* and *Shifa-i Mahmudi*. *Shifa-i Mahmudi* is a translation of *Vagbhatas's Astanga Hrdya*, which directed medical men to put *Unani* medicine on a sound basis, albeit at the behest of the ruling ideology. On the contents of *Tibb-i-Shahabi*, Bernier remarked, "on Physic they have a great number of small books. The most ancient and the most esteemed is written in verse. Their practice differs essentially from ours, and whether these modes of treatment be judicious, I leave to our learned physicians to decide.... I shall only remark that they are successful in Hindoostan."[26]

Royal intervention and encouragement to medical practice assumed a different form when Sikandar Lodi (1489–1517 AD) requested Mian Bhowa, an eminent courtier, to improve healing practices by incorporating useful indigenous drugs and medical practice from *Ayurveda*. The results were seen in his treatise *Madan-ul-Shifa Sikandar Shahi* which highlighted the marvels of *Ayurvedic* medicine,[27] as evident in the following passage:

> By experience, I found that *Unani* medicine did not suit the temperament of the people living in the changed climatic condition of India. Secondly, the names of the medicines were either in Persian or *Unani* (Greek) language, and they were not known to the people of India. Often the *Unani* physicians did not get what they wanted, so there was no alternative except to translate the books of the Indian physicians.

In local and provincial areas, royal patronage had a noticeable impact on the art and practice of medicine. Muslim royalty in the provinces of Gujarat and Kashmir, for instance, encouraged their court physicians to continue composing medical works to promote *Unani* medicine. Ali Muhammad, an eminent physician, was well known for translating works of *Vagbhata* into Persian. Similarly, Mahmud Shah (1458–1511 AD), as part of the Muslim royalty, translated certain *Ayurvedic* works into Persian which was the official and court language at the time.[28] He founded a Department solely for the purpose of translation of medical compilations. Noteworthy translations of this time include *Tarikh-e-Ibn-e-Khallikan*, *Mishkat-Sharif* and *Vagbhata's Astanga Hrydya*. Mansur bin

Muhammad bin Yusuf Ilias, working at the courts of Zain-ul-Abidin (1422–1472 AD) the *Sultan* of Kashmir, achieved fame with his *Kifaya-e-Mujhidya* dedicated to the king. It is evident that several medical treatises produced under the aegis of the royalty were dedicated to their respective emperor, as though to gain royal acceptance. The *Sultanate* period in Delhi offered propitious opportunities for practitioners of the two medical systems to thrive and coexist without one threatening the other. Elsewhere, in the southern regions of India, the art and practice of medicine prospered equally well with the fall of the Bahmani kingdom. The Adil Shahi Dynasty of Bijapur, absorbed by Aurangzeb in later years, is particularly noted for famous surgeons who were "not only encyclopedic scholars of medical sciences, but also skilled artisans,"[29] proving their excellence in the practice of rhinoplastic surgery. The Qutab Shahi Dynasty of Golconda (1495–1686 AD) is known for the publication of the works of two most prominent physicians—Mir Momin and *Hakim*-ul-Mulk Nizamuddin Ahmad Gilani; Mir Momin is sometimes mentioned as a mystic and a holy personality, who commanded respect as a physician at the royal courts, yet was credited with the compilation of two medical treatises—*Risal-e-Miqdaria* and the *Ikhtiyarat-e-Qutub Shaha.* Similarly, Muhammad Qasim in his, *Ikhtiare-e-Qasimi*, for the first time provides a comprehensive account of *Unani* and *Ayurvedic* knowledge based on his personal experimentations and observations. During the successive years, Babur's victory at the Battle of Panipat in 1526 established the Mughal empire. It was the longest rule stretching from the sixteenth to the end of eighteenth century in 1720 with the arrival of Muhammad Shah in India. The period, propitious as it was for medical practice, was marked by an influx of several physicians and surgeons, from Gilan, Shiraz and Tabrez regions in Persia.[30] Extensive interaction between *vaids* and *hakims* was the outcome of professional mobility, encouraging exchange of ideas on pharmacopoeia and therapeutics, and occasionally modifying the scientific paradigm to obtain best results. Such adaptations, Metcalf observed, could not be seen as mere 'accretions' of scientific knowledge because *Unani* medicine demanded adjustments in accordance with the local environment.[31]

Adjustment and accommodation in relation to the Indian environment, and identification and promotion of useful medicinal products through redactions assumed significance when for the first time Hakim Yusuf bin Muhammad, a physician during Babur's reign (1526–530 AD), produced a series of medical compilations integrating the two systems of medicine. He collected relevant material pertaining to hygiene, general principles, diagnosis and treatment of diseases from *Ayurveda* and integrated it with *Unani* medicine.[32] His best works are seen in *Jami-ul-Fawaid* (discussion on chancre), *Fawaid-ul-Akhyar* (benefits of the best), *Qasida-fi Hifz-ul-Sihhat* (preservation on health), and *Riyaz-ul-Adwiya* (garden of remedies). Succeeding his father, Humayun (1530–556 AD) had the challenge of retaining what was bequeathed to him. Success in fighting the invading Afghans in Northern India went alongside his efforts in encouraging medical activities. Several manuscripts on *Unani* medicine were brought out by medical men[33] during his rule. An important encyclopedic work, called *Humayuni*, was compiled by Maulana Muhammad Fazl, a celebrated philosopher-physician at Humayun's court. The work, published in 1539, was based on twelve different subjects, including medicine. After Humayun, Akbar (1556–1605 AD), continued his father's works and ardently supported the cause of medicine. His reign was marked by the spread of *Unani* medicine to every part of India, and the migration of several reputed *hakims* from Persia. Abū'l Fazl, one of the nine gems at Akbar's court, lists at least twenty nine eminent physicians, *vaids* and *hakims*, at the courts of Humayun, including Hakim Ali Gilani, Hakim Abul Fatah Gilani,[34] Ain-ul-Mulk Hakim Shamsuddin Ali Sherazi, Mahadev, and Bhim Datt.[35] Ali Gilani's scientific curiosity and astute observational and clinical skills earned him the royal title of *Jalinus-e-Zaman*, Galen of the Age. He is also credited as the first Indian *hakim* who described the significance of the 'churning' movements of the stomach as a necessary prelude to proper digestion in the human body,[36] and one of the few physicians of the time to look into the histological details of cardiac and other muscles of the body. And by the time Akbar fully established his empire in India, one sees traces of the beginnings of, what Ali calls 'pre-modernization' of India, and of patriotism without revivalism.[37]Akbar promoted both rationalism and social reform through his religious tolerance in later years of his rule. He recognized that India is the birth place of a rich cultural heritage, also seen in Abul Fazl's account of *A'in-i Akbari* which devotes a special section on an '*Account of Hindostan' (Ahwal-i Hindostan)*.[38]

Religious and cultural tolerance, coupled with interest in intellectual activities, marked Akbar's reign as the starting point of the promotion of scientific tradition along with social and cultural developments. It was his quest for knowledge in science and technology that prompted him to support Abū'l Fazl and other men of eminence in his court to make local schools more scientific in their teaching approach. Akbar wanted to see the expansion of science and technology at all levels of school to encourage scientific discussions.[39] He supported the translation of significant works in Sanskrit into Persian, and Persian works into Sanskrit, exemplary amongst which is Bhaskar's twelfth-century monograph on algebra which was made accessible in Persian. Akbar established a Bureau for Translation and Compilation which attracted numerous medical practitioners from distant places.[40] His literary interests included his appreciation for Sanskrit literature which found expression in the numerous Persian translations and adaptations of Hindu epics and other works. These were housed in the imperial library in the city of Agra with a collection of over twenty five thousand books. For such a long era of continued scientific activity and medical writings, there ought to be the personal interest of the rulers, or how else could the medical men gain prominence and earn fortunes. Chandpuri attributes the increasing medical activities to the medical interests of successive kings, and observes that "the spur in the literary activities was the interest that the reigning monarch took in them."[41] For this reason, there were repeated attempts at encouraging medical men to engage in scholarly work at the behest of the rulers. Physicians did well and amassed huge fortunes through private clinics as well as State hospitals. All payments were to be made out of the royal treasury, or *purshigan*. The fiscal strength of Akbar's regime, indicated by the high revenues generated during his time, was another source of monetary support for medical and other scientific activities. Interestingly, medical men of his time engaged themselves not only in medical work, but also in administration. *Hakim* Misri, for instance, reckoned as amongst the prominent men of accounts, was honored as a *mansabdar* by the royal court around 1590s. Known for his medical feats, his success in treating Abū'l Fazl for stone in the bladder and later, Akbar from an injury in deer hunt, won him favors with the Mughal ruler.

The benefits of Akbar's educational activities were not confined to the Muslim population alone. They were also extended to his Hindu subjects through special arrangements for education of Hindu youths in the Muhammadan *madrasas*.[42] Maham Anaga, Akbar's nurse, founded a *madrasa* in Delhi's *Purana Quila* (Old Fort). The quality of education during Akbar's reign is explained in Abū'l Fazl's *Ain-i-Akbari*. The book, completed in 1601, advocates the study of medicine in addition to morals, geometry, arithmetic, astronomy, physiognomy, rules of government and history,[43] thereby suggesting that Indian sciences were not neglected during Akbar's rule.

In order to bring about religious uniformity and stability in his kingdom, Akbar proclaimed the *Din Ilahi* (Divine Religion) declaring himself to be the vice regent of God.[44] This he had hoped would suit both Hindu and Muslim population. In addition to his attitude of religious acceptance, Akbar almost ceased to be a follower of his own faith, and instead constantly revered the Hindu ideal of *dharma*, based on the Hindu principles of performing one's duty. He was led to believe that transmigration of souls was an essential basis of Hinduism, a belief reported by his principal spokesman, Abu'l Fazl who also mentions Akbar's grasp of the doctrine of transmigration of souls and the consequence which such a belief led to in India: divine incarnation not Prophethood. In India (Hind), no one set forth a claim to Prophethood: this is because the claim to Divinity has had precedence here.[45]

An advocate of peace and stability, Akbar believed that equal opportunities for serving the State should be created for Hindus and Muslims alike in order to maintain an empire. It is not surprising that during the course of forty years, Akbar bestowed *mansabs* on at least twenty one Hindus, most of whom belonged to the warrior caste in the Hindu *varna* system, the *Rajputs*. This was also dictated by the Emperor's desire to maintain power over the *Rajput* chiefs who would submit for his suzerainty. The tradition of alliances with Hindu families and nobles through official and personal ties was something Akbar continued from his ancestors which kept the kingdom in a strong position of social ties. His policy of recruitment of Hindu *Rajputs* as Mughal nobles, who were awarded high ranks and perquisites, would have made it easier for Hindu physicians to find employment under the new middle class of nobility. His offer to them of *jagirs* and special administrative offices in his empire enabled *Rajput* chiefs as *jagirdars* to employ local physicians on a more or less permanent basis. On a different level, the co-existence of and common patronage to Hindu and Muslim interests was also reflected in Akbar's interest in Indo-Persian music which he manifested in his 'cultural experimentation by patronizing synthesis and innovation in architecture and painting.'[46] As a 'connoisseur' of vernacular lyrics, Akbar demonstrated reverence for Indian music as mentioned in the vast devotional literature written during the seventeenth century.

With a popular appeal of Akbar's policies of a successful 'synthesis' of all traditions, and his 'eclecticism' of religious experiences,[47] it may seem perfectly logical to surmise that Hindu medicine met the same fate and hence, was not discriminated against under the Mughal regime. This is also exemplified by an almost unimpeachable evidence of support to Indian physicians. Besides the Muslim physicians, three Hindu physicians were appointed at the court of the emperor.[48] This was part of Akbar's policy of reducing the influence of Central Asian nobles who acted like *warrior-grandees* and drew upon inherited positions of power, authority, and influence with their kinsmen. They were heirs to bellicose martial traditions that emphasized personal honor, dignity, and bravery on the field of battle. Always armed themselves, they commanded varying numbers of personal slaves, dependent kinsmen, and paid retainers.[49] Like its scientific counterparts, the science of Pharmacology, as a specialized branch of medicine, also received great attention during Akbar's reign. Most physicians ran private clinics which were open to the people, irrespective of their caste or creed.

The reign of Jahangir (1605–1628 AD) witnessed the worst epidemic conditions of bubonic plague which spread from the northWestern region of Punjab to Sirhind, Doab and Delhi. This called for more intensive efforts to provide medical relief to the people, seen in large number of hospitals established and superintended by physicians for the benefit of the sick. In his decree of *Tuzuk-e-Jahangiri* (hereafter, *TJ*) which was part of his famous Twelve Ordinances, *Ahkam-e-dawazdhagana,* he stated that "hospitals be built in large cities and physicians appointed to attend to the sick; the expenses for this were to be paid from the royal treasury."[50] In his personal memoirs, *TJ*, Jahangir attributed the cause of the epidemic to severe drought from 1613 to 1615. The task of compiling and translating important medical works continued unabated in later years. *Hakim* Ruhuallah, a distinguished practitioner of *Unani* medicine, translated an *Ayurvedic* treatise on hygiene during his reign. He also produced an encyclopedic Pharmacopoeia embodying the techniques and practices followed by *Unani* and *Ayurvedic* physicians for the cure of ailments. Like most of his predecessorrs, Jahangir was well versed in medical science, and carried out various experiments to study the effects of environment on human health. His medical skills and interest, coupled with observational power helped him to prescribe medicines successfully; Jahangir's personal observations on medicine can be found in his memoirs, *TJ*.[51] On the administrative front, Jahangir, although torn between emulation and rejection of his father, inducted disciples "who {are} worthy of receiving *shast wa shabah*. This was the seal or ring and the imperial likeness which were the symbols of disciples."[52]

The Muslim rule was also characterized by the introduction of revenue grants to support individuals and institutions under the aegis of the rulers. These grants, although initiated in the early epoch of Muslim rule, continued to be bestowed by the royalty in later years. As a mark of religious tolerance, for instance, Jahangir proved to be equally liberal towards religious Hindu men, often earning the reputation of a generous king through the several grants he assigned to local religious men. This was done in the form of granting entire village (for instance, Pushkar) in gift, or *in' am*, to the Brahmans of that village. Some *Vaishnavite* priests in Vrindaban were also given new grants in recognition of their divine intellect and work.[53]

The healing art reached its zenith during the reign of Shah Jahan (1628–1658 AD)[54] who took deep interest in equipping the entire country with hospitals throughout its length and breadth, some of which distributed free medicines as part of philanthropic avocation of the emperor. The hospital around the *Jama Masjid* in Delhi, founded in 1650, exemplifies the new move. Shah Jahan also epitomized a rare combination of a statesman and a scientist, and his success as the Mughal grandeur was seen in his efforts at various monumental projects he undertook as part of his move to expand and consolidate the empire. It was in this period that *Hakim* Mashi-uz-Zhaman-Hakim Nur-ud-din Muhammad Abdullah, excelled in surgery and successfully compiled a treatise in 1645, named *Tibb-e-Dara Shikohi*; the treatise embodied the achievements of *Unani* and Indian physicians during the reign of Akbar, Jahangir and Shah Jahan. Equally significant was the work of *Hakim* Amanullah Khan, composed in 1638 to describe the principles of using various drugs and medical practices of *hakims* and *vaids* during the period. Later Mughal period attracted more physicians from Persia. Dara Shikoh, the eldest son of Shah Jahan, had in his court, *Hakim* Ain-ul-Mulk Shirazi, an eminent eye surgeon known for his work on therapeutic drugs, called *Alfaz-ul-Adwiya* (The Vocabulary of Drugs); this work was followed by his *Tibb-e-Dara Shikohi,* attributed to the ruler. In the war of succession between Shahjahan's two sons—Dara Shikoh and Aurangzeb, the two princes appealed to different sets of officials in the imperial administration. While Dara Shikoh's popularity was confined mainly to the nobles, intellectuals and scholars on the same lines as Akbar, Aurangzeb attracted those officials who conformed to the emperor's non-secular policy of fostering Islamic regime; they were the theologians, and Muslim nobles, the *ulema* (Muslim clergy). There is a lot to be said about Dara Shikoh's intellectual curiosity about Muslim and Hindu theological literature. He observed close parallels between the essentials of Hinduism and Islam. So convinced was he about the links that he made them accessible to Hindu and Persian scholars. With the help of *Brahmans* at his courts, he translated the fifty-two *Upanishads* (philosophical texts of the Hindus) into Persian and called it *Sirr-i Akbar*, at the same time translating a Persian work, *Majma'al-bahrayn* (The Mingling of the Two Oceans) into Sanskrit, under the popular title *Samudra Sangam*. His belief in the sanctity of the Hindu *Vedas*, and the *Upanishads* as the ultimate source of monotheism, including Islam, brought an end to his political succession in the war against Aurangzeb in the year 1641. In addition, his almost sacrilegious belief that "no land has been left without prophetic guidance, and that the *Vedas* and *Upanishads* constitute the concealed scripture mentioned in the *Koran,*"[55] intensified the tensions between him and Aurangzeb, and he was condemned to death for his apostasy from Islam and his belief in Hindu idolatry.[56]

The reign of the successive ruler, Aurangzeb (1658–1707 AD) is noteworthy for the publication of most of the standard works on *Unani* medicine. Keswani observes that "it was a highly propitious time for *Unani* medicine to flourish."[57] Because of Aurangzeb's enthusiasm in conforming to a religious polity, unlike his predecessors, he almost confined his patronage to Islamic arts and sciences, and having more Muslim officers in his State employ than ever before. Surely enough, *Unani* medicine and its practitioners formed a significant part of this polity. In doing so, however, the political ethos of his empire and his court culture became more Islamic and less 'eclectic.' He ended the royal patronage to court musicians of previous years. Not surprisingly, "the imperial ateliers were closed and dozens of master painters and their assistants dismissed. Very little monumental building occurred—nothing would match the gardens of Jahangir or the palaces of Akbar or Shah Jahan. Only properly Islamic forms and idioms were encouraged in the arts."[58] Since Aurangzeb withdrew support from chronicle writing and books, it might have had a bearing on the writings and his lack of interest in Hindu arts and sciences. Since only clandestine histories of his reign survive, we cannot be sure that *Ayurveda*, as an 'un-Islamic science,' was throttled by him for if he did, that would certainly have been recorded somewhere, as till Aurangzeb's accession, both the systems were patronized conjointly. Our contention also finds strength in the available literary evidence according to which, various medical compilations of his time have been used by the *Unani* teachers as text books for training students in this field, since 1740.[59] Since the institutions of *Ayurveda* and *Unani* in the late eighteenth century imparted education in both systems of medicine, it is probable that the text books were utilized by *Ayurvedic* teachers too. Many local wealthy elites financed the founding of hospitals where *Unani* and *Ayurvedic* physicians could be employed to continue working on medical compilations; the most famous compiler of Aurangzeb's rule was *Hakim* Muhammad Akbar Arzani. In 1650, Aurangzeb funded the establishment of a hospital in Delhi, superintended by prominent physicians. It may appear that medical practice would not have survived but for the royal patronage it received. The following section will, however, prove that the Muslim royalty had a special motivation in perpetuating the interests of a special class of people, the middle classes, who as the chief beneficiaries of imperial grants became a succor to the two medical systems.

Revenue Grants and Middle Classes: Patronage outside the Royal Courts

Royal support to medical systems made it propitious for medical practice to prosper under the aegis of the rulers. It is evident that patronage consisted in encouraging physicians to develop medical literature and in establishing hospitals and clinics where *Ayurvedic* practitioners could work in collaboration with *Unani* physicians. One can surmise then that *hakims* and *vaids* and other professionals, and merchants constituted a distinct category of social groups in *Mughal* India—distinct because, their means of sustenance were independent of feudal property.[60] The physicians at the royal courts obtained a respectable income and the salaries earned would be characterized as feudal patronage[61] rather than for a service in demand.[62] This was true of the physicians serving the State in Mughal India; a majority of the former was Persian. These were generally more prosperous and enjoyed greater social prestige.

Of the several revenue grants in Mughal India, there were some assigned for the maintenance of medical schools or *madrasas*, set up in the late medieval period as centers of education in the field of *Unani* medicine. The grants, often referred to as *auqaf,*[63] were assigned permanently in trust for the maintenance of the institutions, including *madrasas*, religious shrines and tombs. They were also used for the subsistence of their staff, and for charities disbursed through them.[64] The grants, once assigned, gave the emperor the privilege to determine how and by whom it was to be managed. As an example, Akbar, who made the initial grant of 18 villages to the shrine of Mu'inuddin Chisti at Ajmer, not only decided the issue of succession of the spiritual head of the shrine, but also appointed its *mutawalli* (administrator).[65] As for its Indian counterpart, there is no evidence suggesting that the Mughals proscribed *Ayurvedic* medical schools. In all possibility, given the progressive work environment, *Ayurvedic* practitioners did equally well in their practice along with *Unani* physicians. Unlike in previous years, the practice of surgery, thus, did not face any opposition from the ruling ideology. On the contrary, royal patronage to medical practice spurred the growth of medical knowledge, hitherto unknown in ancient times.

Revenue grants, known as *imlak*, were a characteristic feature of the Mughal rule in India. They were introduced by Akbar so that he could alienate his right to directly collect the land revenue from a specific area of land. Officially, these grants were better termed as *madad-i ma'ash* (aid for subsistence), which were instituted primarily for the "maintenance of the poor and indigent (creatures) of God."[66]

The best source providing a detailed description of the various grants conferred is Abu-l Fazl's, *Ain-i-Akbari*; Abu-l Fazl was a minister to Akbar and a renowned historian during Akbar's reign. The book mentions four groups of people to whom the grant was given as a special privilege. These excluded men who ere engaged in any trade or service or had a means of sustenance, and included men in higher learning, divine men (Brahmans), people of noble lineage who would not accept any employment, and finally, people who had no means of earning a livelihood.[67] In effect, men of learning and devotion were the prime holders of the *madad-i ma'ash* grants, although few of them also went to Muslim women (from the erstwhile Persia). It is believed that Jahangir appointed a foster-sister of his father, Akbar, to take charge of grants to Muslim women for learning and religious devotion.

An interesting feature of the system of allocating grants and alienating grantees for the purpose was the existence of other groups of men who did not fall in any of the categories listed by Abu-l Fazl. One such group consisted of physicians treating the poor and the infirm within a local region, and received special grants, as evidenced in a series of documents relating to Gujarat. Records also show that the *Mehervaid* family of *Parsi* physicians of Navsari in the State of Gujarat was conferred the grant issued by royal decree, *farmans*, of 1664 and 1702.[68]*Meher* denotes a *Parsi* personal name to which was added *vaid* to indicate their medical profession so that in later years it became *Mehervaid* or *Vaids* of *Meher* family. Interestingly, *Mehervaid*, the founder of the family, practiced Indian medicine, and had made this a life time occupation so that even later members became successful hereditary medical practitioners. In some instances, *Mehervaid* members practiced medicine as a philanthropic avocation by establishing charitable clinics and dispensaries for the poor infirm. Impressed by this, Akbar also granted them a *jagir* (special honor for services) near Navsari along with financial support for personal maintenance of practitioners to the extent that Navsari became synonymous with *Mehervaid* family and its medical practice. In addition to plasticizing *Ayurvedic* medicine, some of them supported *Unani* medicine. This is supported by the names of *Mehervaid's* father, Sayer, and grandfather Kamdin referred to as Tabib.

Holders of *madad-i ma'ash* had the right to collect the land revenue, and were exempted from paying any land revenue which meant that they could keep the revenue they collected. Despite these privileges, however, no provisions were made for the heirs to grantees who had to apply for a renewal of the grant. It was not until 1690 when Aurangzeb, for the first time, issued a *farman* which made the *madad-i ma'ash* hereditary, and declared, "the land of the imperial grantees, conferred by valid *farmans*, old and new, would be retained, completely and fully, without loss or reduction, by the heirs of the deceased grantees, generation after generation."[69]

Support outside the royal courts created a new class of physicians. There were physicians of the lower echelons (or ordinary physicians) who belonged to the class of *vaidyas*,[70] and were supported by the middle classes of *Mughal* India, the *mansabdars*,[71] and the *jagirdars*[72] and in some cases, holders of the *madad-i ma'ash* grants. The latter appointed them as consultants looking after the health of the troopers, and offered them handsome perquisites. This created more attractive opportunities for *tabibs* (*hakims*) from smaller towns to seek employment under the *mansabdars*.[73] In some situations, even the local *jagirdars* could also allocate a small portion of their land tax-free to give away in return for services to them, even though it was meant to last till the duration of the assignment. It is possible that these services could well be provided by medical practitioners for we know that the latter had the support of the middle classes. Some of the State-established towns also offered employment opportunities to physicians at the lower echelons. Since the latter were assigned the task of caring for the troopers, their services were considered equally indispensable for the efficient functioning of the imperial war machine.[74] Holders of *madad-i ma'ash* grant, over a period or time, created a class of people who ceased to devote any time to religious learning, for which the grant was originally intended, and instead depended on land as a permanent source of living. Available evidence indicates that some grantees "freely acquired *zamindaris* and even acted as revenue-farmers."[75]

The successful expansion of the Mughal empire in the rural areas relied upon a special class of men, the *gentry* class, who occupied prominent positions in the local economy, prominent enough to sustain the Mughal agrarian structure. The literate trading castes of the *gentry* class, also called *mahajans*, provided another area where medical practitioners could seek their fortune. For they were part of that administrative structure created by Akbar which "intruded beneath the tough defenses of rural life and reshaped the economy, culture and society of Mughal India."[76] Akbar controlled these grants held by Muslim theologians to extend them to non-Muslim population, but by doing so, he created conflicting situations with the holders of the grant who later became groups of special interest by Jahangir. He called them *Army of Prayer* in appreciation of their services as being indispensable to the royal military army. And when Aurangzeb acquired royal power, he made the grants hereditary, although some of them in Sher Shah's reign were held to be conditional. For instance, the historian and theologian, Abdul Qadir Badauni, received a grant in the form of a land, for which reason he was obliged to provide military services for the kings, and maintain a small cavalry contingent for the army.[77]

Given the above changes in the economics of Mughal India, one is faced with the challenge of understanding the role played by that section of the society which constituted some form of 'non-feudal property rooted in the money economy.' This section comprised the middle classes which became "formidable competitors of the *jagirdars* and *zamindars* for exercising control over the peasant communities."[78] Primarily, they represented the non-feudal stratum of society comprised of the mercantile class (the merchants, *sarrafs* or money-changer, banker) and *mahajans* (money-lender), and the urban intelligentsia of professional and service groups. Khan[79] provides an impressive account of how these groups came to represent a 'distinct social category' of the non-feudal property in Mughal India. He dwells on the lack of clarity on classifying the nature of payment made for services to the urban intelligentsia as part of the feudal property, seeing it as an income in return of services offered to their clients. However, in the sociological parlance of the definition of 'specialized skills as property taking a different form,'[80] the income of the specialized services to the kings and nobility would be characterized as a form of non-feudal property. Although it is difficult to ascertain the exact income they obtained for these services, there is little doubt that there was a great demand for which reason some of the middle class professionals like clerks, accountants, physicians and teachers amassed huge fortunes for their services.[81] The character of nobility during the later years of Shah Jahan's reign changed when not only *Rajputs* but Turanis, Indian Muslims, and Afghan *amirs* (nobles) were addressed as *khanazad* (one born to the house). The term implied more of a familial and hereditary service to the emperor, than an emotional connotation. Although the *khanazads* retained their sense of devotion and sacrifice to the ruler, they considered their nobility as a prerogative which made their character different from that under the previous rulers. They were, however, loyal and possessed qualities necessary for a royal political acceptance. Bhimsen Saxena, a *mansabdar* belonging to the *Kayastha* caste, and portraying himself as a *khanazad,* wrote a memoir indicating the extent of the ethos of service that had pervaded in subordinate technical officers. As Bhimsen writes, "the *Mughal* emperor was the true servant of God and his agent who tries to foster peace and prosperity. The fruits of the empire were human happiness and well being."[82] The two levels or classes of physicians, one working with the *mansabdars* and the other serving the kings and nobles, gave a new character to the practice of medicine during the Mughal period. The lower echelons of the State would employ physicians in the imperial war machinery to look after the health and take care of the wounded in war situations. Because of the significance of the nature of services provided under the *mansabdars*, it was not surprising to find local physicians moving to bigger towns and cities for employment, and quite often, the physician seeking employment "was already having considerable clientele in his own locality."[83] In terms of the nature of services offered, there was no disparity, and although the former outnumbered those at the State level, their services were considered on par and hence, equally significant. On this score, Moreland[84] thinks that since the demand for medical services was low amongst the society at large, physicians and private medical practitioners could only hope to survive on the services offered to the high ranking officials in the feudal hierarchy, the kings and the nobles; the income, thus received would be seen in terms of feudal patronage. His view on the low demand may be not be entirely true because we know that some of the physicians did very well and became rich, especially in the northern part of India. The following passage, compelling as it is in its argument, should prove the obvious in this respect.

> We come to know from a casual remark attributed to *Pir Hassau Teli* that towards the beginning for the sixteenth century, services were available of private practitioners in the market places of Lahore... There is also a specific reference to *Hakim Basant* who practiced at Lahore during Shahjahan's reign. He is mentioned in connection with the illness of the wife of a petty official who was under *Hakim* Basant's treatment for some time. An idea of the wide demand that existed at Lahore for medical services during Aurangzeb's reign can be had from the *Manucci's* memoirs. After his service in Dara Shikoh's artillery ceased abruptly with the defeat of that prince, he established himself at Lahore as a private practitioner. The first person whom he treated successfully was the wife of a *quazi*[85] who had been given up as a hopeless case by all Persian and Indian physicians. This made him very popular among the nobles as well as the 'lower order.' So great was my name that I had of being fortunate with the cases that I undertook, writes *Manucci*, that they came from many places distant from Lahore to call me in to visit patients. It seems that *Manucci's* income from his private practice at Lahore was much greater than what he could hope to earn in the service of a noble. When Muhammad Amin Khan, the governor of Lahore, offered to employ him as a physician, *Manucci* politely declined the offer since he considered the proposed salary insufficient.[86]

In view of this, it seems that State patronage was not an absolutely essential factor for indigenous medical system to thrive during the period. Instead, physicians working with the new middle classes did fairly well, though not as well as those at the royal courts.[87] The question now is who were these middle classes? Were they a part of the Mughal royalty or were they created as a result of the special privileges offered to them in return of their services to the royalty. The answer lies partly in both.

Under Muslim rule, the middle classes included various categories of revenue officials holding high positions in the central and provincial governments during the fifteenth and sixteenth centuries. Throughout the Mughal period, there existed a great demand for medical services, especially in places like Jaunpur, Banaras, Hissar, and Delhi where some private practitioners earned a considerable reputation, often hired and paid for their services. In addition, there were also some 'lesser known' practicing physicians who remained dependent on private practice to earn their livelihood, although some of these were believed to be no better than 'quacks.'[88] Available evidence suggests that the lesser *tabibs* also served various officials at the provincial level and country side. In Hissar (in modern Punjab) for instance, during Aurangzeb's reign, a local physician, Manka *Tabib* won accolades and amassed huge fortunes through his expertise in pulse examination.

It seems evident that there existed in the Mughal empire, a demand for medical services at various levels. It may also seem that given different levels, there would be a hierarchical base in the nature of services provided. But that was not the case. Although physicians serving the kings and nobles enjoyed greater social prestige, there was no difference in the quality of the services provided. In terms of social prestige and honor, the Mughal emperors valued attributes of merit and learning for which reason they would often grant *mansabs* to professionals in recognition of their services, or may even raise them to the status of nobles. This also helped to maintain long-term ties with the nobility in the expanding phases of the empire. For instance, Jalaluddin Muzaffar Ardistani Hakim Alimuddin, and *Hakim* Daud were entitled as Wazir Khan and Taqarrub Khan, respectively, aside from their positions as nobles. The truth was that together they constituted a distinct and an 'exclusive clientele' of medical practice under the Mughal regime. More specifically, they included the petty officials, merchants, traders and the urban intelligentsia.[89] One question that looms large at this stage is how did physicians at the two levels receive their training? It might be safe to assume that the medical men at local levels received their training from the court physicians or at the State-sponsored schools. Many of them were trained locally and practiced medicine in their local community. Also, several *hakims* and *vaids* passed on their knowledge to their sons in the traditional atmosphere of *madrasas*. In some cases, their clinics and homes served as centers of education for a close didactic atmosphere. The existence of different echelons of physicians also allowed a fair degree of mobility from the local to the State level which made physicians at the lower echelons autonomous of the royal court. In the long term however, contradictions, and the ensuing wars during the eighteenth century proved egregious for the patronage system of medicine.

Decline of Mughal Power and Agrarian Crisis: Dwindling Clientele and Dwindling Patronage

During the late Muslim period, there set in a gradual deterioration and fragmentation of economic and political stability in the Mughal regime when conflicts began to develop at different levels of bureaucracy. The nobility, which earlier had played an important role in the institutionalization, expansion and consolidation of the Mughal rule in India, saw itself disintegrating following the death of Aurangzeb. Thus, the Mughal rule, while it created a sense of unity and showing progress in the fields of art, architecture, sciences and technology, also declined as a result. Several reasons have been forwarded for the collapse of the centralized bureaucracy in Mughal India. They ensued over the *zamindars*[90] share in land revenue or surplus produce. Also, the restrictions imposed on the *jagirdars* by the Mughal emperors, the exploitation and maltreatment of the peasant mass and the *zamindars*' inability to exact high revenues from the peasants, eventually challenged the Mughal authority, and led to a revolt against the imperial administration. The revolts of the early part of the eighteenth century "marked an assertion of the power of local 'despots' against the Mughal system, and perhaps were symptomatic of a kind of social resurgence."[91] Gradually, the *jagirdars* and *mansabdars*, who were the chief agents for collection of revenue, found themselves at odds with the stringent policies of the Mughal bureaucracy, which meant that sometimes their inability to extract the economic surplus proved inimical to their social position in the system. In addition, the *jagirdar* had to conform to the imperial regulations of governing his *jagir*.[92] The assignments of a *jagir* formed the main source of income for the Mughal empire. There was no fixed period for which the *jagir* could be held; it was normally held by the same person for not more than two or four years.

For the peasant mass, the usual way of expressing their disagreement over these measures was through armed resistance. Quite often, the army was led by *mansabdars* with *jagirdars* as their support, and the aristocracy lived "as it did from grants paid directly out of the imperial treasury, or from the dues paid by peasants on the *jagirs* granted by their masters in the empire, to maintain their rank."[93] The situation became more intense when a series of famines ravaged the country at the time, thus aggravating exploitation of the peasants. As a result, most peasants were unable to pay high taxes which compelled them to migrate to neighboring regions—thus, peasant migration remained a central feature of agrarian life in Mughal India. In the seventeenth century, the system of *jagir* transfer worsened the economic burden on the peasant mass, which heightened and became more apparent when during Aurangzeb's reign, his *farman* of 1665 declared a disproportionate increase in the amount of revenue—disproportionate in relation to the produce of the land. As a result, the *jagirdars* felt compelled to exact more revenue from the peasants. The burden of payment on the peasant population became severe to the extent of affecting their daily survival. And when the *raiyat* (peasant) was unable to pay the revenue, he was "beaten unmercifully and maltreated."[94]

In order that the peasants do not cease to pay the revenue, and to safeguard their own interests, the *zamindars* did not apply the rules and regulations imposed by the authorities, and hence gained more support from them. They also demanded a larger share in the land revenue or in the surplus produce from the emperor. The two, thus, became associated in a joint struggle against the Mughal administration, often expressed as an armed conflict. This sets an example of the middle classes being antagonistic to the State under the Muslim rule, with peasant participation in major revolts against the Mughal regime. Even the local *nawabs*,[95] *jagirdars* and *mansabdars* began to exercise their autonomy by increasing their revenues and profits. In addition to an increasing burden on the peasant masses, there were sporadic incidents of maltreatment of Hindus by the Mughal rulers. Despite the internecine conditions prevailing at the time, the practice of medicine remained uninfluenced. For it had the support of the *mansabdars* and other social groups in the social strata of Mughal regime. Under these conditions, the number of physicians serving the royalty began to decline after Akbar so much so that even amongst the the existing few, most practicing physicians were of Persian origin. Abul Fazl, Badauni and Nizamuddin Ahmad mention the existence of about thirty nine physicians (14 Persian, 12 Indian and 13 others) at Akbar's court, reduced to 11 (7 Persian, 3 Indian, and 1 amongst the category of others) under the reign of Shah Jahan.[96] The medical systems suffered a decline when its patrons—the State and the middle classes—vanished with the gradual consolidation of the British empire in India. In any case, the number of Persian nobles recruited by Akbar to serve the expanding needs of his empire began to decline in later years of Mughal rule. This meant that the support base of physicians provided by the nobility also had begun to shrink. Coupled with this were contradictions in previous years which resulted in rebellious actions by various social groups. The result was take-over by a new imperial administration. The victory of Robert Clive at the Battle of Plassey in 1757, the invasion in 1761 by the Afghans, and the victory of the British over the Portuguese and the Dutch were strong enough to dismantle the Mughal empire, hitherto under a state of flux. The period also witnessed a severe time for the upper classes when the British, having acquired greater control over Indian society, disregarded the village as a revenue-paying unit only to "press upon the upper elements that had so far been favored with lower rates."[97] Gradually, the smaller *muqaddams*,[98] of the *mahalwari* [99] system, and the *mirasdars*[100] of Bombay, the kingpins of old communities tended to be leveled with the lower strata of peasantry.[101] There was also a subsequent decline in the urban employment of troopers, retainers and servants. The latter were actively supported by the Muslim regime and the middle classes or, in Habib's words, "the previous appropriators of the surplus."[102]

Both ancient and Muslim periods, thus, were characterized by a centralized authority with the State at the helm of all activities, including medical and scientific activities. In both cases we have seen how the ruling ideology and the State played a major role in creating or sometimes even stifling the progress of medical knowledge. The difference, however, lay in the existence of economic surplus under Muslim rule. This means that in order for a scientific or medical activity to sustain within the social fabric, economic surplus, be it directly with the rulers, merchants or dispensed through the central authority or the State, is essential for it to thrive well.

The downfall of the Mughal sovereignty after Aurangzeb did not hamper the spread of medical art in the country, although the relations between the emperor and the nobility and senior officers had became severe as a result of Aurangzeb's rigid expressions of new policies. He supported the notion of *khanazadgi* rather than discipleship to define this relation, which became a weakness in the Mughal political ideology in later years. Nevertheless, later Muslim rulers continued their support for the expansion of literary activities, even if it meant success at a different level from previous years. *Hakim* Mohammad Sharif Khan became the pioneer of *hakims* and of *Unani* medicine, earning fame for his family of patrons of medicine, while *Hakim* Ajmal Khan is associated with the foundation of the *Tibbia* College in Delhi. Throughout the post-Mughal period from 1719 to 1828, physicians compiled several compendia based on translated medical terms, and wrote commentaries of their observations and clinical experiments. For the emperor, the usual way of recognizing their work was to provide incentives by conferring specific titles of honor. Shah Alam II (1759–1806 AD), for instance, conferred the title of *Ashraf-ul-Hukama* on *Hakim* Muhammad Sharif Khan, a physician at his court who was granted a *jagir* in recognition of his works, *Ilaj-ul-Amraz* and *Tuhfa-e-Alamshahi.*

It seems apparent that the existence of the medical traditions outside the royal courts was made possible by the patronage they received from the nobility and the lower echelons of the feudal system, despite the latter's conflict with the State. Besides, the 'non-royal' support (in terms of the new social classes), there were other factors that facilitated the co-existence of *Ayurveda* and *Unani*. After all, *Unani* medicine was not indigenous and successfully merged with its Indian counterpart under the Muslim rulers. Briefly, these factors concern similarities in their focus on compilation work, on the manner of dissemination of scientific knowledge and on the scientific basis of humoral theory.

Ayurveda and *Unani*: A 'Blissful Bond'

Common patronage at the royal courts and by the middle classes under the Muslim rule was facilitated by parallels and similarities between *Unani* and *Ayurveda* so that one system did not threaten another. These included focus on writing medical compendia, sometimes at the behest of the rulers, the manner in which medical knowledge was imparted for professional training, and a similar basis of disease diagnosis and therapeutics.

Literary Achievements

The period of Muslim rule in India witnessed the foundation of several clinics by eminent physicians who were given grants to compile theoretical achievements in medical practice in the form of medical compilations. The focus on literary activities embodying the healing art was so great that it seems that the medical practitioners, as Zahuri[103] asserts, had made it a practice to gather their life-long experiences in book forms to present as a gift to the reigning personages. Their experiences embodied various modes of treatment, their effects, and qualities of herbs and medicines on various diseases, their uses, which were often presented as comprehensive compilations of medical experiences; patients' condition and medical history were essential topics of study. The period was, thus, marked by an increase in the number of compilations,[104] perhaps mistaken for new scientific achievements. The physicians carried out experiments on locally available medicinal herbs to assess their efficacy as therapeutics, and the succeeding generations of these made additions to what their ancestors had left. The literature on *Unani* medicine, thus, continued to grow unabated.[105] Adding Kuhn's notion of scientific change,[106] the physicians, instead of attempting to solve puzzles (or medical problems in this case) which, in turn, would have led to a more explicit articulation of the paradigm (that is, the traditional medical system), were occupied with compilation and literary work with a few noticeable additions of new therapeutic agents based on their experience. Although there was continuity and spur in the literary sphere, there was no significant breakthrough or discovery which would have necessitated the re-strengthening, let alone replacement, of the older paradigm to assimilate these new concepts and beliefs. If success were to be judged by paradigmatic changes, then it might be logical to argue that medical practice of earlier periods was confined more to adding to the theoretical base of medicine, and less to major scientific revolutions or breakthroughs. This was true for both *Unani* and *Ayurveda.* The latter, though emerging as a science in the sixth century BC, was reduced to compilation work by its practitioners in later years; original texts were redacted by several learned men who remained occupied with increasing the indigenous pharmacopoeia through literary writings.

The above account indicates the similarity in professional work in the two medical systems—that of an increase in the number of medical texts, with an increase in the *ad hoc* accretions with no identifiable paradigmatic break in medical arguments.

Professional Training

Two systems of training existed during the ancient period in India—the Brahmanic system, and the formal institutionalized system of education, or the Monastic system. The Brahmanic system emphasized medical training through generations, not by formal institutions or colleges but through individual training by a skilled practitioner; the latter belonged to the priestly caste regarded as an infallible authority. This system of imparting medical knowledge was prevalent in the *Vedic* period when the entire society was dominated by the privileged class, the Brahmans and the priests who possessed the undisputed right to learn the *vedas.* The Monastic system, on the other hand, involved training through universities, as seen during the time of Buddha.[107] Several Buddhist works mention the existence of the Monastic system. For instance, *Jivaka*, a contemporary of Buddha, received his education at the University of Taxila, under the preceptorship of *Atreya.* The system was successful as a training system in the post-*Vedic* period when there medical training had to altered subsequent to a change in the methodology of medical science from magico-religious to material and scientific outlook.

A similar shift in the manner of disseminating scientific knowledge was observed in *Unani* medicine during the rule of the Muslims. The practice of medicine in early Muslim rule was, many a time, a family occupation. That is, the knowledge of medicine was transmitted from the teacher to the student who invariably happened to be his son.[108] It was, thus, practiced through generations from father to son, as is also evident from the many families of *hakims* whose successors even to this day are engaged in *Unani* practice. One such genealogy of *hakims* is mentioned in a medical text entitled *Imtihan-ul- alba-le-quafat-il-al- tiba.*

In the later years of Muslim rule, especially during the reign of Akbar, several people came to India to study medicine under the noted physicians to the king. Evidence suggests a series of descendants or heirs of physicians practising *Unani* medicine in some clinics during the Mughal period for four to five generations continuously.[109] It is also known that initially, there were no established schools of *Unani* medicine, and each *hakim* trained students in medical learning in a personalized didactic atmosphere; the physicians' clinics facilitated as centers of education. It is possible that the new outlook on medical facts based on a synthesis of the two systems of medicine, called for a more formalized system of training young aspirants in the field.

Referring back to the halcyon days of the healing art under royal support, Firoz Tughlaq and later Mughal rulers evinced keen interest in financing medical schools, in addition to regular *madrasas*, to develop medical education.[110] Regular institutional training, however, began in 1883 with the founding of *Madrasa Tibbiya* by Hadiq al-Mulk *Hakim* Abd al-Majid Khan,[111] in Delhi. Other schools and institutions for higher learning in *Unani* medicine followed the trend which confirmed parallels in training practices of disseminating medical knowledge in the two systems.

Common Base of Medical Practice

The theory of body humors, which occupied a central place in the diagnostics and therapeutics of *Ayurveda* and *Unani*, facilitated the co-existence of the two medical traditions. Practitioners of both viewed proportions and balance of body humors to conditions of health and disease; imbalance or disturbance in these resulted in the impairment of health. The humoral theory of *Unani* medicine supposes the presence, in the body, of four humors—blood, phlegm, black bile and yellow bile, each possessing a particular quality of heat, coolness, dryness end humidity, called the temperaments. The drugs utilized by *Unani* medical practitioners are classified according to the body temperaments in restoring the original equilibrium of body humors. Diagnosis was successfully done on the basis of pulse examination, and any prominence or pulsation of blood vessels was taken as a pathological symptom. In *Ayurveda*, body functions are regulated by humors, recognized as air, bile and phlegm which formed the basis of the trihumoral theory. Based on the ancient Greek medical concepts of Hippocrates, *Unani* medicine developed the tetrahumoral hypothesis. The two medical systems, thus, had parallels in terms of imparting professional training, the emphasis on compilation work by physicians and medical scholars, and lastly, the therapeutics based on the humoral theory. Given the nature of literary activities under Muslim rule, the period was distinctly characterized by proliferation of medical compendia as the only and major achievement under the ruling ideology and the nobility. It was as if the entire literary work was dedicated to the reigning personages so that "*hakims* of various parts of India produced a large number of books on the various branches of medical science on the basis of *Unani* or *Ayurvedic* medicine and on the basis of their experience of medical cases."[112] This may have been a sequel to lack of regular institutional training during the period which otherwise would have necessitated empirical observation and analysis of scientific data. Even for *Unani* medicine, the system of education and training centered on the preceptor-student relationship which entailed training in a closed didactic atmosphere. Education in the homes or clinics of physicians did not require discussions and scientific dialogue between the teacher and his pupil, and hence limited the infusion and exchange of new ideas. Since the Greek concepts supported by Arabic medical scholars were recognized as 'unassailable' by *Unani* physicians, it is not surprising that the *hakims* throughout the period maintained the status quo of the medical theories contained therein. For this would have challenged the very basis of medical practice, otherwise believed to result from several years of dedication by scholars. The only way in which the pristine medical culture could be treasured was through medical compilations and commentaries which often remained theoretical in nature.

Conclusions

It is logical to conclude at this stage that *Ayurveda* received royal support not only from the ruling kings in ancient times, but also accepted patronage from the Muslim rulers. In fact, it may have fared better in this period and even more so during the later Muslim rule after the introduction of special grants and the support of middle classes. State patronage to *Ayurveda* in previous centuries can also be gauged from the achievements its practitioners made, especially under the Gupta kings for which the period if often regarded as the 'best era of Hindu medicine.' Nevertheless, the period was also marked by continuity in redaction work by eminent physicians, translation of important *Ayurvedic* works and the several encomiums brought by *Vaids*, under royal and middle class patronage.

It is apparent that the peaceful co-existence of *Ayurveda* and *Unani* during this period was not always because of State patronage; it was more a result of the internal similarities between the two systems so that one system did not threaten another. And since *Unani* medicine had been a part of indigenous pharmacopoeia for several centuries, it could easily merge with the scientific activities of *Ayurvedic* physicians. Also, despite State support, the practice of medicine was confined to compilation work. This is not to disregard the usefulness of medical writings but to suggest that given its nature, medical science was unable to win accolades with new discoveries or for major scientific breakthroughs. Three levels of support to medical systems are discernible at this stage. These include the royal support, the support from middle classes, and the internal similarities between the *Ayurveda* and *Unani* which facilitated a 'royal' and a middle class compensation and common patronage to the two systems. The fall in grace of the practitioners of indigenous medicine, however, was a consequence of the collapse of the Mughal empire and the subsequent liquidation of their patrons at local levels, represented by the middle classes and the nobility. The deterioration of the Mughal army was a result of the gradual disappearance of Mughal nobles who sought fortune and fame under the Mughals in later years. After all, signs of such a decline really began soon after Akbar's policy of 'India for the Indians' which facilitated an easy association of Hindus with the imperial administration, and hence a decline in the entry of foreigners into the country; it was apparent that the influx of men from neighboring countries provided better opportunities for the Mughal emperors for recruitment to the royal service. Conflicts in the Mughal administration almost seemed to be a corollary of the decline in the military nobility which threw prosperous physicians into a state of chaos and a period of uncertainty. This suggests that it is not so much the lack of State support but the lack of a strong clientele base, albeit outside the confines of State support, which is crucial for a larger understanding of the character of medical art and practice.

Reflecting back on the period prior to the Muslim rule, it was apparent that the ruling religious ideology proved inimical to scientific development which the practicing physicians of the time tried to evade by offering 'ransoms' or religious concessions to the rulers. Notwithstanding the earlier opposition to *Ayurveda*, the tradition was accepted by the State and by the orthodoxy in later years. The subsequent period of Muslim rule, witnessed the acceptance of the two medical traditions by the State. In the case of *Unani,* particularly, there is no evidence of an incorporation of religions or magical elements. The Mughal period, in particular, never exhibited much predilection for 'ethnic, natural or class exclusiveness.'[113] The nobility of Babur and Humayun proves this point. It included Iranis, Turanis, Uzbeks and Afghans—even though for political reasons, the Uzbeks and Afghans, were considered the chief enemies of the Mughals. There were a few Indian nobles at the Mughal courts, but they were either converts to Islam or descendants from West and Central Asia.[114] In the absence of major scientific breakthroughs, historians of science would despair at calling medical profession in India fully professionalized. But it might still be too early to make any pronouncements on the state of medicine during the Muslim rule, or even to assume that medical practice had become stagnant by this time. In doing so, there is no intent at dismissing or doubting the level of medical achievements of earlier medical men. The validity of our argument can only be seen after a careful consideration of the status of medical practice in the following period of British rule, which is the focus of our next chapter. The British period is prticularly made more interesting by the introduction of Western or bio-medicine by the British. The 'stagnation' became apparent with the dynamic character of Western medicine, and while the new concepts of Western medicine were recognized, indigenous science still prevailed as a body of knowledge 'waiting to be re-discovered' in the optic of its Western counterpart. The following chapter will discuss the curious interaction between Western and Indian medical systems which, by the time of British entry, represented a 'syncretic' medical tradition of *Ayurveda* and *Unani.*

Chapter 4

Colonial Imperatives, Medicine and Indian Response

> We are informed that there are in the Sanskrit language many excellent systems of Ethics, with codes of laws and compendiums of the duties relating to every class of people , the study of which might be useful to those natives who maybe destined for the Judicial department of Government. There are also many tracts of merit, we are told, on the virtue of plants and drugs, and on the application of them in medicine, the knowledge of which might prove desirable to the European practitioner, and there are many treatises on Astronomy and Algebra, which, though they may not add new light to European science, might be made to form links of communication between the natives and the gentlemen in our service, which are attached to the Observatory and to the department of engineers, and by such intercourse the natives might be gradually be led to adopt the modern improvements in those and other sciences.[1]
>
> —Court of Directors, Public Disputations

Amidst the general chaos and conflict of the sixteenth century following the death of the last Mughal ruler, Aurangzeb (1707), the autocratic base of the Mughal army deteriorated, and the empire collapsed. In the absence of a centralized authority, the country was in political and social decline, and became an arena of political struggle among the Mughal successors, the Persian adventurers, the Afghan leaders, the Marathas and the Sikhs; between 1748 and 1762, the country saw a civil warfare with repeated invasions by the Afghans. It was this civil warfare which led to the disappearance of the Mughal nobles. Most importantly,

> within little more than a decade after *Aurangzeb*'s death, seven fierce battles for the imperial succession occurred, in which large numbers of princes, nobles, and trained soldiers were slain, while armed hostilities between leading nobles re-

> sulted in further waste of superior man-power. The *Nizmu-l mulk*, for example, was forced to battle with three rivals in order to secure the viceroyalty of the Deccan; the struggle for the Governorship of Gujarat was marked by three fatal contests. The loss of life resulting from these internecine feuds was augmented by the mortality caused by punitive operations against the Sikhs and the Marathas.[2]

The warfare and an inequitable economic system also impoverished the revenue-producing class under the Mughal rulers. Although Bahadur Shah I tried to establish peace after Aurangzeb, the final blow to Mughal sovereignty came from Nadir Shah, the Persian ruler who went to India 'for loot than for conquest.' He sacked Delhi and returned to Persia with the *Kohinoor* Diamond and the Peacock Throne.[3] As a result, the internal political and social situation of the country weakened, thus making it vulnerable to occupations by the British and the French. The European incursion into India had already begun in the fifteenth century when Vasco da Gama established the Portuguese empire in his zeal to seek Christians who could help him in his crusades, and spices to control trade in spices in the East Indies. As part of expanding trade activities, the British established the East India Company in 1600, a chartered commercial enterprise dealing with trade in silk, gems, spices and indigo. In 1608, the Mughal Emperor had given the right to the Company to establish a trading post in Surat in the Western part of India. It was after the Battle of Plassey in Bengal on 23 June 1757 that the British emerged as the major power, making Bengal the first seat of political and social control over a society whose social fabric had become dilapidated as a result of dissolution of stable polity.

British Dominion and Western Medicine

Looking back at what the Mughal rulers left behind as an outcome of their policies towards medical sciences, it is clear at this stage that with the Mugha*l* ascendancy over India, *Ayurveda* was never looked down upon. Practitioners of *Ayurveda* and *Unani* collaborated with a similar paradigmatic approach in an environment that facilitated mutual exchange of medical ideas. As Basham remarks, "whatever the *ulama*[4] and the Brahmans might say, we have no record of animosity between Hindu and Muslim in the field of medicine."[5]

The Battle of Buxar of 1764, between the *nawabs* (princes) of Bengal, Oudh, the Mughal emperor, Shah Alam and the British, was the real foundation of British dominion in India, although the Company rule ended in 1857 with the transfer of power to the Crown. By the time the British gained political hold in the country, traditional institutions and customs were confronted with "the most subversive of ideas—about justice, administration, philosophy, politics—and were to be transformed, in some cases superficially, in others fundamentally, by the impact of the West."[6] An immediate result of this confrontation was displayed when the British introduced their Western medical science in India. Indian medicine, by this time, represented a syncretic body of medical knowledge, comprising both *Ayurveda* and *Unani*, which Leslie calls 'traditional-culture' medicine because it included *vaids* and *hakims* whose practice was modified by changes in the new methodology of empiricism and later commentaries and oral traditions.[7] So what happened to *Ayurveda* during British rule in India? The near unanimous pronouncement is that Indian medicine declined as a result of the introduction of Western medicine by the British. But did it really stagnate, or was it because of the alternative system of medicine brought by the British with its dynamic scientific potential that *Ayurveda* for the first time was seen as stagnant?

It is commonly believed that the British not only rejected *Ayurvedic* medical system,[8] but also disregarded the health of the civilian population. However, that may not have been the initial British reaction to *Ayurveda*. It is is also accepted that the British opposition to *Ayurveda* stems from the imperialist hubris, hegemony and political control—a fact, which cannot be easily discounted. Accepting this view with no explanations or cogent reasons, might lead to analytical distortions at this stage. Hence, it will be appropriate to consider factors which may allow one to understand more comprehensively the considerations that went into the possible downgrading of *Ayurveda* by the British. These additional factors concern the initial, and growing differences between the development and practice of British-borne Western medicine and indigenous medicine. It will be seen in the following discussion that despite these differences, indigenous medicine thrived well and was accessible to a large Indian population. This was an outcome of a series of political events that changed the way the Indian population, the practitioners, and the clientele of Indian medicine viewed indigenous medicine vis-à-vis its Western counterpart. Added to these changes were the British policies and the manner in which the colonial administrators evaluated indigenous medical knowledge during situationf of competition from keen enthusiasts and proponents of *Ayurveda*.

Initial Encounters: State and Indian Practitioners

By the early years of the nineteenth century, the East India Company had adopted a general attitude of 'indifference' and non-interference with Indian society. The British administrators realized that popular acceptance of any undertakings were indispensable to preserving peace in the country, and that any attempts at interfering with either religion or traditional customs would subvert Companies' policies. This attitude was clearly displayed in the medical policies implemented at the time. Indifferent, as they were initially, there was an element of accommodation of local practitioners who were trained in indigenous medicine. They employed Indian physicians as subordinate health workers in hospitals manned by British physicians.[9] Those attaining professional skill working with the latter were later attached to regiments and civil stations as *Native Doctors*.[10] When the East India Company recognized the scale on which it had to govern the country, it expanded its scope of medical activities to include indigenous healers. This belief was strengthened when Company officials started believing that local diseases were best treated by local doctors–a view prevalent throughout most of the eighteenth century.[11] In order to translate this into practice, the Company also hired local people as its assistants and gave them elementary training in Western medicine.[12] At this stage, limited medical knowledge of the Western world in handling issues of public health and sanitation inspired Western physicians and administrators to make best use of available expertise. Evidence shows that indigenous physicians were employed by the British as early as 1690 and by the year 1762, the Company had employed as many as nineteen *Native Doctors*. As part of the expansion of medical services, Leslie[13] notes that the *Native Doctors* were trained in Western medicine at the Civil Hospital in Calcutta. Some *vaids* also found employment with the Company in the Madras Presidency. According to Crawford, Indian practitioners were also employed on the cruisers of the Bombay marine in the beginning of the nineteenth century. While medical training of *Native Doctors* figured high in the list of colonial medical policies, Western medical institutions were expanded to accommodate more Indians to be trained as apothecaries.[14] By the second half of the nineteenth century, with the expansion of the British rule and of British society as a result of increase in new administrators in the country, there prevailed a sense of 'superiority' over the Indian population. After the Mutiny of 1857, there were tendencies to reform the Indian society, especially at a time when "the British in India had virtually institutionalized their contempt for things Indian."[15]

The Charter Act of 1813 which extended the Company's rule until the next renewal twenty years later, ended its trade monopoly in India, but paved the way for allocation of annual funds for education. Learning about the local culture formed a significant part of this venture. The first such attempts were best seen in 1814 when the Court of Directors in London expressed their desire to investigate the medicinal value of local indigenous plants, by experimentation as well as by studying ancient texts of medical learning. Gradually, the increasing demand for native practitioners, coupled with the appreciation of the *Ayurvedic* treatises in Sanskrit language by the Court of Directors of the East India Company, created a congenial atmosphere for the establishment of a separate medical school. In 1822, the Company laid the foundation of a school for *Native Doctors*, called the *Native Medical Institution* (*NMI*) in Bengal.[16] The institution represented the first organized effort by the government for the communication of medical instructions to the natives[17] in indigenous and Western medical sciences. The indigenous part of the medical curriculum was taught in Indian vernaculars of Sanskrit and Urdu. Starting with a modest twenty students, The *NMI* had registered over fifty students by the year 1826. Students trained at the *NMI*, were, according to the then Governor General, to be appointed in the Native Corps.[18]

Indian medicine and its practitioners then did well under British regime, and in 1824, a Sanskrit college was established at Calcutta where instructions in medical science were given through the medium of Sanskrit. In 1827, more teachers were appointed to lecture in Sanskrit to students of *Ayurveda* and to acquaint them with the works of the eminent medical authorities—*Caraka, Susruta*, and *Vagbhata*. The medical curriculum included parallel instructions in Indian and Western medical sciences; rudimentary treatises on anatomy, surgery and medicine were made available in Indian vernaculars to facilitate combined teaching of Western and Indian textual knowledge.[19] The initial move to encourage the two systems jointly was short lived which paved the way for radical reforms in educational policies in later years.

End of First Synthesis: Abolition of the Native Medical Institution

Of the several factors that led to the abolition and demise of the *NMI*, James Mill's *History of British India* remained largely influential in providing a direction to British policies. Mill's work, which he wrote in 1819 when hired as Assistant Examiner of Correspondence at the India House in London, provided the basis of most social and cultural policies in British India. His utilitarian thinking inspired Thomas Babington Macaulay to project an India based on English culture. Mill's controversial, yet deeply powerful, book coupled with his attitude of distrusting Oriental despotism, was akin to Lord Cornwallis' Native Exclusion Act of 1791 which excluded Indians from all higher government positions in the imperial machinery. Despite an overt condemnation of all Oriental people, and anti-Asian undertones, the work served as a basis for most policies in colonial India.

The Cornwallis era (1786-1793) may be looked upon as a westernizing interlude between the genesis of Orientalist cultural policy of Warren Hastings and the extension of that policy under Marquess Wellesley. It is interesting how in all policy matters, Lord Cornwallis chose alien solutions to Indian culture problems, defining what was best in English administrative machinery.[20] Hastings, on the other hand, wanted to "produce an elite of acculturated Englishmen."[21]

Mill's influence on cultural policies in India proved inimical to the growth of favorable policies for the Indian population. Thus, in 1828, when William Bentinck went to Madras as the new Governor-General, he arrived with 'Mill's-like' anti-Orientalist cultural policy, communicating to Mill, "I am going to British India, but I shall not be Governor-General. It is you that will be Governor-General."[22] It is no wonder then that the entire Bentinck era, although often viewed as an extension of British reformism in India, remained highly disruptive for Indian intelligentsia who were lost in the cultural crisis of their society. The growth of cultural institutions almost became stunted under the administration of

William Bentinck. For instance, the College of Fort William was dismantled and ceased to exist in 1834 in accordance with Charles Trevelyan's decree justifying its abolition. Other institutions followed suit. The Asiatic Society became burdened by financial crisis. Most importantly, educational institutions like the Calcutta *Madrasa* and Sanskrit College became close to being non-existent. These events became the precursor to the Orientalist-Anglicist controversy in later years. They also gave a chance to the older generations of Indian intelligentsia to institutionalize their protests in defense of Hindu duties, way of life, and culture—first through the *Brahmo Sabha* (Organization of God) in 1828, and later through the *Dharma Sabha* (*Dharma* or way of life, *Sabha* or organization) in 1831. *Brahmo Sabha* acquired a religious basis with Ram Mohan Roy's puritanical 'return to the *Vedas*' view in defense of the *Vedic* golden age, while the latter was formed in recognition of Hindu way of life and culture.[23]

In 1835, Lord William Bentinck appointed the Public Instruction Committee for the purpose of enquiring into the conditions of medical education and training in India. His ideas of governing the country drew largely from the general climate of evangelical thoughts in England which sought to modernize India through the benefits of Christianity. The Committee was charged with the task of suggesting measures that would be expedient to adopt with a view to the better instruction of the people, including the arts and sciences of Europe. The Committee summarized the defects of the *NMI,* and argued that it was not properly organized. It complained that the tuition, period of training and examination in *Ayurvedic* medicine were inadequate and that courses on practical anatomy were non-existent. In 1835, in accordance with the Committee's suggestion, William Bentinck passed an order announcing the abolition of the institution. Medical classes at the Sanskrit college were discontinued in the same year.[24] Bentinck's order also decreed that a new College be established for instructing Indians on the pattern adopted in Europe and that instructions be given through the medium of English which replaced Persian language and became the business and official court language of India. This alteration in the medium of instruction also followed Macaulay's vehement attack that the content of higher education should be Western-oriented and that the language of instruction should be English. This meant "the end of the first attempt at synthesis of the Eastern and Western systems of medicine in India for the benefit of the Indians; this also ushered in an era of political patronage and recognition of the Western systems of medicine."[25]

Viewed as an assault on tradition and indigenous modes of thought, the move was enough to engender a reaction amongst the Indian nationalists, and cultural enthusiasts who made several attempts at resuscitating *Ayurveda* by political propaganda and by institutional support. Their efforts found expression after provincial governments were set up to assess and support the efficacy of indigenous medical traditions [26] in later years.

Initial support and reverence for indigenous medical knowledge changed in the years following 1835 when British policies focused on pushing indigenous medicine out of their agenda in order to patronize teaching and practice in Western sciences.[27] Despite this shift, the popularity of *Ayurveda*, especially in rural areas, inspired colonial administrators to employ indigenous practitioners as part of their plans to extend medical relief. Indian practitioners were employed through various schemes introduced in different parts of the country, and one such scheme was introduced in Punjab in 1867.[28] Yet another clue to the recognition of *vaids* and *hakims* comes much later, and is provided by the 1938 Act of Bombay which gave the indigenous practitioners the same rights as the Western doctors;[29] the former were employed to extend medical services in rural areas. Since the first three decades of the twentieth century were rife with several political and cultural changes in response to British rule, concessions for utilization of indigenous physicians may well have been under pressure from Indian nationalists.

During the late nineteenth century, the proliferation of Western medical schools and colleges made the benefits of collaboration with the British and their education system more visible and accessible to the indigenous population. The fact that training in Western medicine ensured the Indians a State-recognized status and better chances of entering into the service of the State, the railways and the like, also indicated a changed attitude of the British to Indian practitioners. Indian physicians trained in indigenous medicine, on the other hand, found it difficult to compete with their counterparts from the elaborately-equipped colleges of Western medicine, that gained popularity as a result of monetary support for scholarships and distribution of free medical books for its publicity.[30] Better prospects of seeking employment after training in allopathic or Western medicine were enough to inspire the orthodox *vaids*, previously averse to studying medicine, to send their sons to colleges of Western medicine. Despite an emphasis on the study of anatomy and surgery which, otherwise would have offended the established caste prejudices, the higher castes of Bengal, especially Brahmins, were found to comprise a majority of the students at a college of Western medicine in Dacca.[31]

Indian physicians during British supremacy were then categorized into three classes. Students trained in Western colleges were designated as First-Class *Native Doctors*; those trained in the short-lived *NMI* founded in 1822, and still another category of physicians trained in hospitals, were enrolled as Second- and Third-Class *Native physicians*, respectively.[32] The existence of different classes of physicians gave rise to a series of new bureaucratic statuses occupied by practitioners of indigenous medicine, some of whom gained knowledge of European medicine with what Leslie[33] calls, various degrees of eclecticism. These physicians possessing a knowledge of Western medicine claimed a superior status to other indigenous practitioners as a result of which conflicting tendencies developed between orthodox Hindus and *vaids*, the former amongst whom practiced *Ayurveda* as a philanthropic avocation but increasingly adopted medicine as an occupation.[34] The conflict often turned severe when certain *Ayurvedic* physicians claimed to be English doctors administering 'English medicine,' with no training or familiarity with the tenets of Western medicine.[35]

Surviving the Odds: Indigenous Medicine *sans* Official Patronage

While Western medicine gained a firm footing in colonial India, indigenous medicine did well with the support of an indigenous clientele in the form of indigenous practitioners as well as patients. The former were healers, and their descendants amassed huge fortunes through grant of land in recognition for their services by the Muslim royalty, but they lost these privileges when the British reduced the income of the royalty. It was this group of practitioners who fell from their grace, and hence from loss of elite patronage and joined the growing middle-class market for medical services under colonial rule. Jeffery[36] sees this decline in the status of indigenous practitioners and their science as becoming apparent between 1860 and 1920 when they began to establish new institutions to promote and publicize indigenous medicine. Not surprisingly, they also "began to emulate aspects of Western medicine, not merely because the British institutions had a higher prestige and state backing but also because market conditions for indigenous medicine permitted this kind of occupational organization."[37]

Despite the increase in the number of colleges of Western medicine, Indian medicine continued to be taught and practiced in the traditional manner. Practitioners of *Ayurveda* trained young aspirants in their homes called *Tols*. The local population generally continued to profess faith in indigenous medicine, and often preferred a *kaviraja* or *vaid* to an allopathic doctor. After 1835, although British policy was to supplant traditional systems with their own, Indian medicine drew local clientele as its patrons. The founding of the *Native Medical Society* in 1832, with the object of confining medical practice to *vaidyas* alone, is the earliest record of the association of indigenous practitioners,[38] which diverted them from acquainting themselves with European medicine. Indian medicine continued to have a willing support of the *Native Medical Society* of indigenous practitioners and local clientele.

Two names draw our attention when we discuss the status of *Ayurveda* in the post-1835 era with the official declaration of patronage to Western sciences. They were Gangadhara Ray (1789–1885) and Gangaprasad Sen (1824–1896), leading *kavirajas* belonging to a family of reputed physicians. Gangadhara Ray, credited with his contributions and patronage to Indian medicine in British India, trained several students in his *Tol* at Berhampore in Bengal Presidency, and wrote Sanskrit commentaries on *Ayurvedic* texts; the most famous was *Caraka's Jalpakalpatyaru*.[39] His junior contemporary, Gangaprasad Sen of Calcutta also contributed to the preservation of the traditional medical knowledge, and is credited as the first person to export indigenous drugs to Europe and America, as a move to promoting *Ayurveda*. Realizing what might get the attention of people, he emulated some of the professional traits of Western medicine by introducing a consultation fee, and advertised the efficacy of indigenous at fixed prices, thus diverting 'popular attention' from its Western counterpart.[40] The two physicians trained an illustrious generation of *vaids* who practiced in different parts of Bengal Presidency.

It is clear that the establishment of medical colleges in accordance with those in Europe could not supplant indigenous medicine, which continued to thrive under the patronage of indigenous practitioners. In 1929, Bills were moved in the Legislative Assemblies to expand financial aid in setting up schools and colleges of indigenous medical systems. Not surprisingly, issues on the employment of *vaids* and *hakims*, and pecuniary aid to institutions of indigenous medicine were a consistent theme in the municipality boards and government institutions.[41]

Alongside continued efforts by indigenous physicians to seek financial support for indigenous medicine, there was also a gradual acceptance and acknowledgment of Western medical knowledge, especially toward the second decade of the nineteenth century. Indian physicians established and funded several *Ayurvedic* colleges with the idea of including Western medical science in the curriculum. These efforts were best seen in the foundation of the *Gobinda Sundari Ayurvedic College* in 1922 by *Kaviraj* Ram Chandra Mallick, and the *Vishwanatha Ayurvedic College* in 1932 by *Kaviraj* Gananath Sen, in order to modify practical aspects of indigenous medicine. In 1878, Indian physicians opened a dispensary in the Calcutta and propagated knowledge of Indian medicine through inexpensive books on the same.[42] They highlighted the importance of *Ayurvedic* pharmacopoeia, and founded several pharmaceutical concerns to manufacture and sell indigenous drugs. This, however, enabled the *kavirajas* to earn considerable wealth so that they were at one time, what Gupta[43] claims "among the richest men in the country."[43]

Indian Medicine Revisited: Changing Attitude of the British

It is possible that *Ayurveda* was looked down upon by the British simply because of imperialist hauteur. However, as medicine is itself such a practical body of knowledge, hauteur must rest on some very practical considerations if a body of knowledge dealing with such a crucial area as health is to be looked down upon, and almost proscribed. In ancient times, religious interference proved inimical to medical progress, and although the orthodoxy may have attempted to downgrade *Ayurveda*, it did not banish it. It is also known that some of the renowned ancient *vaids* were patronized by the royal courts. But if in British India, *Ayurveda* was not considered to be a suitable and reliable medical compendium of knowledge, then did the British have an alternative? Of course they did. But was the alternative such that it exposed *Ayurveda* as a defunct or at least a stagnant system of medicine? The argument here is that it probably did and this gave further ammunition to fuel and rekindle the basic cultural hubris that most imperialists exhibit. In contrast, the abolition of the *NMI*, however, did not always mean a total exclusion of Indian science. Between 1887 and 1898, there were repeated attempts by the colonial administrators to utilize skilled indigenous practitioners and train skilled *hakims* and *vaids* as a move to extend medical relief to the population.[44] The favorable attitude of the British toward Indian medicine and its practitioners can be attributed to two reasons; firstly, the end of the nineteenth century was a turbulent time for the prevailing social and political situation in the country. The nationalist movement by this time had gained a strong hold in its struggle against colonialism, and the British made sure that they did not implement a policy which would aggravate the political crisis. Secondly, the British wanted to fill the void in medical services which could not reach the vast Indian population. This then was imperialist tolerance and accommodation at its best.

Judging by the competitive propensities within the two medical traditions, it may be reiterated that the ancient theories, on which the *Ayurvedic* system of medicine was based, little coincided with the knowledge of the British for which reason the system did not carry much favor with the Europeans.[45] But this is not to label *Ayurveda* as wholly unscientific, and according to Leslie, the indigenous medical system involved a rational use of naturalistic theories to interpret empirical observations and also utilized efficacious methods for promoting health and curing illness. But if judged by other criteria such as the standardization of techniques or the employment of sophisticated experimentation methods, the system, perhaps, made apparent the inherent differences in medical practice.[46]

It is important to note that Indian surgeons had a lot to offer to the corpus of medical practice at a time when Western sciences were shedding their garb of supernatural beliefs as a result of scientific and industrial revolution in Europe. Indian doctors were known for their remarkable feat in performing surgical operations of the nose, called rhinoplasty. The first operation was performed in 1792 on Minocher Cowasjee who had his nose cut off when taken prisoner by *Tipu Sultan*. The entire operation was witnessed by Thomas Cruso and James Findlay, who were amongst eminent medical men of the time.

What then were the reasons for the denial of political support to *Ayurveda*? Indian medicine was at times labeled as 'quaint' by the advocates of Western medicine. As a sequel, several proposals in favor of establishing *Ayurvedic* colleges were rejected as impracticable and in 1926, the possibility of claiming a superior or even an equal status for the indigenous systems of medicine, in surgery, bacteriology, parasitology and research in general, was ruled out by the

British administrators.[47] The decision was also based on the belief that Western medicine was founded upon an accurate knowledge of anatomy, physiology and pathology for which reason it was suggested by Sir Pardey Lukis, the then Assistant Surgeon of Burma, that *Ayurvedic* system must sooner or later be superseded by the medical system of the West.[48]

Differences between Indian and Western forms of medical knowledge became obvious in the area of medical education, the medium of instruction and the level of scientific knowledge and use of scientific instruments, which diverted colonial policies towards Western medicine. Historians would despair at the veracity of this argument, for it is accepted that the denial of official support had a history of political events which culminated in viewing Indian sciences as different and possibly, 'inferior,' to European sciences. Nevertheless, an allusion to some of the differences will be useful at this stage.

Indian and Western Medicine: Professional Rivals?

The discipline of ancient medicine was, by and large, similar in most countries where medical knowledge developed in association with their cultural heritage. The practice of dissection for purposes of anatomical knowledge, in general was lacking or even prohibited by the ruling authorities in most ancient civilizations. In the late nineteenth and early twentieth centuries, however, medicine moved a step further when it made significant strides in medical knowledge which altered the style and efficacy of medical practice. These discoveries included development in the use of scientific instruments, advances in anatomy, surgery, especially in the field of gynecology and obstetrics, and the development of nosology.

Medical Technology, Anatomy and Surgery: Indicators of Medical Progress?

The medical system of the eighteenth and nineteenth centuries in the Western world had its origin in the early Middle Ages of Europe when two developments characterized the literary medical tradition: the growth of a stratified medical practice, and the rise of specialized medical institutions, medical organizations, guilds, public doctors, teaching institutions. These trends were parallel to the urbanization of European society and culture which became apparent after 1050 AD.[49] Western medicine, when it came to India, represented a literary tradition which had undergone radical changes in the sixteenth and seventeenth centuries. Medical practice had begun to be characterized by the use of instruments, which enabled a more acute form of diagnosis. By these instruments, qualitative judgments could be broken down to manageable quantitative measures allowing greater reliability and uniformity in both teaching and practice. For instance, prior to the thermometer, diagnosis was purely qualitative[50] in that the state of a patient was described as *feverish*, and changes in the state accordingly labeled him as less *feverish* or more *feverish*. Similarly, other oft-used instruments like the minute-watch, the stethoscope and the microscope helped significantly in the development of Western medicine. The significance of these instruments is not seen in terms of discoveries but also to the extent they helped the practicing physician to diagnose and categorize ailments more effectively.[51]

Alongside the use of newer instruments, anatomical and surgical studies had a major influence on the practice of medicine. Anatomical studies which gained prominence in the fifteenth and sixteenth centuries, provided a new perspective of medical practice when physicians sought to rely heavily on performing dissections to further their knowledge of disease.[52] Paracelsus was known for his fight against orthodoxy and achievements in medicine, and Vesalius for raising the scientific status of human anatomy based on direct clinical observations. What Paracelsus did for medicine, and Vesalius did for anatomy, Ambroise Pare (1510–90) did for Renaissance Surgery. His anatomical writings on raising surgery to a professional stature revealed his success in performing surgical operations in war situations, as well as treatment of fractures and dislocations. Added to this was his position as an army and military surgeon and association with the French kings and their troops which earned him the title of 'Father of Surgery.' The period was also marked by the development of techniques of amputation and the method of treating fractures by Francois Chopart (1743–95). One might argue that for long, even in the West, the study of anatomy and practice of dissection were not part of the medical curriculum. These were carried out in the halls of barber surgeons who insisted on their prerogative of dissecting human bodies. Dissection was regarded as a "punishment, a fate worse than death, even while it was serving the purposes of medical knowledge."[53] Although, Jean Francois Fernel's work on the significance of physiological and pathological experiments in the early decades of the sixteenth century made anatomical studies indispensable for diagnosis of diseases, surgery and dissection of the corpse continued to be held in low repute on moral grounds. In Europe, dead bodies could be opened up for research purposes, "sometimes for coroners to peer inside to discover the 'truth' of death."[54] In France, this was given more meaning when "the public did not consider it permissible to open up the secrtes of the body for such purposes."[55]

Moral restraints in dissecting corpses and the difficulties in procuring them for research purposes changed the perception of corpses in medical circles. By the seventeenth century, corpses became a 'commodity' when bodies "were dismembered and sold in pieces, or measured and sold by the inch."[56] In Britain, the need for surgeons was always on the increase, especially in the early nineteenth century. Besides, the rapidly increasing population was not proportionate to the number of surgeons available. The need was partly met by the establishment in 1800 of the Royal College of Surgeons, and also by providing a new focus in medical curriculum. The ghastly practice of stealing corpses from graveyards became widespread, and so did the manner in which these were purveyed to medical researchers for dissection. But the practice came to an end first with the foundation of a Surgical Society by Charles Hastings in 1816, which demanded strengthening the professional status of doctors, and second with the Anatomy Act of 1832 allowing a lawful acquisition of bodies.

Problems did not, however, end here. Issues of an increasing rivalry between apothecaries, as trained in handling medicinal dugs, and untrained grocers, who claimed the same status as apothecaries, caused serious controversies in the medical circle. The solution lay in altering the content of training which would justify their respective status. Thus a five-year apprenticeship including clinical experience in anatomy and physiology formed a necessary prelude to the licensing of apothecaries. It is possible that the shift in the focus of medical training making clinical expertise as indispensable to medicine, may have led Bentinck to order a revision of medical education in India, not long after the Act came into force. Since medical education in India did not include study of anatomy, due in part for the same prohibitions as in Europe, it gave an opportunity to the British to substitute Indian medicine by European medicine. But we know that medical ideas and discoveries which constitute modern day medicine, already existed in Indian medicine thousands of years prior to the advent of the British. In anatomy, in particular, Wise argued that "the Hindus were the first scientific cultivators of the most important and essential of all the departments of medical knowledge, practical anatomy."[57]

During this period, surgery changed its approach to handling individual cases and a new dimension of handling diseases, so that by the end of the nineteenth century, it dominated the hospital business. The changing needs of medical practice in nineteenth-century Britain called for an increased establishment of hospitals as institutions for the care of the sick. They also represented "Britain's entrepreneurial nature in its first century of industrialisation."[58] In this changing medical environment, the field of women and their specific health problems for the first time gained recognition with the series of intra-abdominal operations performed by Ephraim McDowell (1771–1830). Prior to the mid-nineteenth century, physicians either refused to examine or took little interest in women, irrespective of the nature of their affliction. McDowell's first ovariotomic operation in 1809, however, introduced a new chapter on caring for women with specific health problems. By the latter part of the nineteenth century, James Marion Sims won accolades for his successful operative treatment of vesico-vaginal fistula,[59] thus opening up a new field of study in the health problems of women which earlier had received little or no attention in the medical world. He also founded the first gynecologic hospital, Woman's Hospital, in the State of New York in 1855. Robert Lawson Tait's emphasis on sepsis added a new perspective to ovariotomic operations in the second half of the nineteenth century. The discovery of anesthesia and antisepsis allowed surgeons to perform more ambitious operations.

Obstetrics was another branch of medical science which became more sophisticated in its use of medical technology over a period of time. Earlier, the practice of obstetrics had been the work of mid-wives. But development in the type of instruments and techniques of obstetrical operations required the expertise of surgeons specialized in the field. Hendrik Van Deventer (1657-1721), a leading obstetrician of the eighteenth century, successfully conducted a study on the variation of the female pelvis and their effect upon labor. Similarly, the benefit following the work of John William Ballantyne (1861–1923) on antenatal pathology, and his pioneering efforts in establishing clinics for the care of the expectant mothers and the unborn child, proved incalculable to the medical profession.

The growing emphasis on post-mortem examination facilitated diagnosis by disclosing the structure and relation of various parts, and by contributing to anatomy and physiology and secondly, by exposing the real site of the disease, thus rendering safer the methods of treatment and making prognosis more accurate. In other words, study of morbid anatomy facilitated the quest for effective methods of combating diseases. This was an important contribution of anatomical studies to Pathology and Pathologic anatomy, pioneered by Giovanni Battista Morgagni (1682–1771). Morgagni demonstrated the importance of localized image of disease to medical practice when he described various forms of tumor and lung diseases through autopsy dissection,[60] and gave detailed descriptions of carcinoma in the liver. The importance of clinical histories, thus, came to be considered indispensable for autopsy results in identifying the exact nature of the disease. Study of pathological anatomy was gradually enriched by the subsequent work of Marie Francois Xavier Bichat (1771–1802), also known for founding the science of histology. Bichat's discovery was an improvement upon the previous work by Morgagni with the transfer of the site of diseases from organs to body tissues. Further advances in medicine were the result of the systematization of a new area of study, cellular pathology, in 1855 by Rudolf Ludwig Carl Virchow. Based upon scientific research, cellular pathology not only dominated biology and pathology but also replaced the much acclaimed old humoral theories.

Nosology was another branch which altered the manner in which Western physicians viewed disease situations in the eighteenth century through a systematic classification of diseases. A great exponent of the new progress was Thomas Sydenham (1624–89), an English physician who dismissed previous theories as inexplicable, embarking on studying a natural history of diseases. His theories were supported by John Locke (1632–1704), a philosopher, who also believed that "the acquisition of medical knowledge was being thwarted by hypothetical systems concerned with providing the hidden causes of diseases."[61] He was one of the first to prescribe iron for the cure of anemia, and the first to popularize the use of cinchona bark in the treatment of ague or malaria, a disease prevalent in eighteenth-century England. Later in 1714, attempts at classifying diseases were continued by Fernel and thereafter cellular pathology and bacteriology opened up new developments in the medical field.[62] Attempts to systematize diseases received a great impetus in the middle of the eighteenth century following Linnaeus' classification of plants. Though he was not a medical man, he created a similar classification of human diseases.

The development of nosology and pathology, gradual as it was, thus ushered in a new style of diagnostics and treatment. Defining individual diseases based on objective symptoms of the disease at the sickbed, marked a significant change in the physicians' search for specific cures. Nosology helped to separate victims of one kind of disease from another; differentiation of measles from scarlet fever provides a good example of this, and this also helped in containing infectious diseases to a great extent. The abandonment of the theory of *fevers* revolutionized the art of Western medical practice, not only by enabling Western physicians to specify different kinds of ailments, but also in the search for different treatments for what was hitherto considered a similar affliction. To this effect, physicians in their search for improved therapeutics, moved from mere theoretical basis of diseases to bedside for detailed observations of clinical symptoms. So much for this new development. In *Ayurveda,* as in other ancient medical traditions, the science of nosology was rudimentary, if not primitive,[63] and this marked another great divergence between Western and indigenous medicine in both theory and practice. Disease situations were dependent more upon the internal imbalance of the body humors than on external factors. Since bacterial infections did not find a place in these theories, germs in *Ayurveda* were considered ubiquitous. Thus, when Robert Koch announced his discovery of the *vibrio* of cholera in 1884 and his idea of its transmission by drinking water, it helped and inspired many facets of research in prevention, control and therapeutic aspects of the disease. Overwhelmed by this discovery, Edward Jenner claimed, "may I not with perfect confidence congratulate my country and society at large on their beholding an antidote that is capable of extirpating from the earth a disease which is every hour devouring its victims; a disease that has ever been considered as the severest scourge of the human race."[64] His pioneering work on vaccination as a means of prevention of disease enabled the medical profession to score almost total victory over several other infectious diseases.[65]

Inoculation against smallpox, initiated in Britain, spread rapidly in the second half of eighteenth century. Inoculation, introduced on a mass scale at the turn of the twentieth century also helped to control small pox. It was also responsible for making possible successful efforts in eradicating the anopheles mosquito, the carrier of malaria, thus making a considerable impact on the native population. The period between 1870s and late 1880s also witnessed the development of new discoveries in Western science. Louis Pasteur's work attenuating bacterial cultures paved the way for developing new vaccines and antitoxins. Although this was a laboratory 'accident' in 1879, it revolutionized medical thinking about disease by changing the concept of 'killers' to 'benefactors.'

Impact of Medical Advances: Medical Training Re-Assessed

The imperial administrators took the dynamic character of Western medical science as a 'mirror' to view similar developments in Indian medicine. And because Western medicine portrayed itself as a source of legitimacy offering systematic explanations of phenomena in terms of cause and effect, it imposed limitations on the efficacy of its indigenous counterpart, demanding scrutiny of the latter's scientific essentials. This called for a re-assessment of the medical training then existent in British India. One such institution which became an object of scrutiny was the *NMI* which, as discussed in previous sections, was abolished in 1835. It will be useful to look at the compelling reasons for the recognized differences between the two medical traditions in terms of medical training.

The first formalized training in British India[66] dates from 1812 prior to which European surgeons had trained assistants on an apprenticeship basis, some of whom had later been recruited to subordinate medical services.[67] The manner of disseminating knowledge of ancient medicine was one of an intimate relationship between the teacher and the taught in the *Tols* of *kavirajas*, or *vaids*, where the only medical topic taught was internal medicine or drug therapy. This did not call for training in clinical aspects of medicine. In contrast, instructions in Western medicine were given in hospitals and dispensaries established by the British. Though there was a steady growth in the number of colleges of medicine, modeled on the ones in England after 1835, initial training in hospitals incorporated important aspects of practical and clinical instructions. For the British, medical education was 'defective' with no clinical focus. The characteristic 'defect' of *Ayurveda* incapacitated *vaids* from being on the alert for new diseases and new remedies or modification of therapeutic measures. At least the British thought so.[68]

During the rule of East India Company, William Bentinck, who was recalled as the first Governor-General of Bengal in 1828, arrived with a philosophy which was "openly anti-thetical to Orientalist cultural policy."[69] Mill's controversial *History of British India* won him a key position as a policy maker in the East India Company. With a low esteem of Asians and 'Oriental people,' Mill reinforced his thinking through Lord Cornwallis' (Governor General) Native Exclusion Act of 1791 which stated that

> even in manners, and in the leading parts of the moral character, the lines of re-sem blance (between Indian and Chinese) are strong. Both nations are to nearly an equal degree tainted with the vices of insincerity; dissembling, treacherous, even in manners, and in the leading parts of the moral character, the lines of re-sem blance (between Indian and Chinese) are strong. Both nations are to nearly an equal degree tainted with the vices of insincerity; dissembling, treacherous, mendacious, to an excess which surpasses even the unusual measure of uncultivated society. Both are disposed to excessive exaggeration with regard to everything related to themselves. Both are cowardly and unfeeling. Both are to the

> highest degree conceited of themselves, and full of affected contempt for others. Both are in a physical sense, disgustingly unclean in their persons and houses.[70]

Mill developed a critical view of Indian society as backward and stagnant. The members of the Public Instruction Committee appointed by William Bentinck were divided in opinion on whether education in general, was to be imparted in European languages, or according to Indian vernaculars. The former, called the Anglicists, demanded that the Company replace all traditional learning by education of the West. They were part of the pressure group of the Radicals who believed in the superiority of the Western world. The second group, of the Orientalists, wanted to promote indigenous education, at the same time were sensitive to Indian susceptibilities in traditional norms. Gradual reform, if necessary, seemed the most obvious instrument of appeal to the Indian population. The controversy was settled in favor of the Anglicists of which Thomas Babington Macaulay was the most vehement protagonist. In 1829, in a letter to the government, it was made clear that the admitted policy of the British government was to render its own language gradually throughout the country.[71] Bentinck also stated that the chief aim of the educational policy should be to promote a knowledge of European literature and science, and that all the funds appropriated for the purpose of education would be employed in imparting education in Western literature and science through the medium of English. Surprisingly, despite the controversy and the subsequent introduction of English as the medium of instruction in all European arts and sciences, there was never any discussion or attempt to study and report on the educational progress according to indigenous system of education. Indigenous education was often considered inconsequential, and because of lack of written sources on the subject, the only evidence from which one can draw inferences on the educational progress in pre-colonial India is the Reports by William Adam (on Bengal, 1835-38), Mount Stuart Elphinstone (on Bombay, 1823), and Thomas Munro (on Madras, 1822).[72]

Oriental learning was ridiculed and, perhaps, considered inferior to Western learning, as is clear from Frazer's[73] remark that the historical information which had been collected from the books written in Sanskrit language was less valuable than what was to be found in the English texts. The considered supremacy of English language and the over-riding importance attached to English literature and science by its advocates prompted the British to discontinue classes in 1835 when they decided to substitute the entire system of education by the one adopted in Europe. Bengal, in particular, saw an irate reaction from the Orientalists and Indians who argued that the achievements and contributions by the Hindus were too well-founded to be dismissed in 'so trivial a manner.'[74]

The insistence on English as the medium of all recognized forms of knowledge in itself incapacitated indigenous forms of medicine or science from attaining acceptance and recognition. By making English as the medium of instruction, the British made it well-nigh impossible for training in indigenous medicine to follow a format that would meet their approval. This then was imperialist hauteur at its best. But it is also possible to argue that the British could have made an exception in the case of *Ayurveda* if the science of *Ayurveda* had appealed to them, in which case the British policy on the medium of instruction was based on the belief that Indian medicine had nothing of consequence to offer them. This is probably an overstatement, but the vast gulf between *Ayurveda* and Western medicine, got wider everyday so that by the turn of the twentieth century many Indians too believed that it could not be breached.

These developments and discoveries contrasted sharply with Indian medicine and it was the immense advances which appealed to the Indian population for which reason *Ayurveda* began to lose its clients.[75] At this stage, descendants of local elites, who were in close alliance with the British during the early part of nineteenth century, also moved away from Indian medicine. The Registration Act of 1912 limiting the entry of indigenous practitioners, seemed to threaten the enormous clientele base of *Ayurveda*, with almost 90 percent of the population dependent upon indigenous medicine. The amicable existence of *Ayurveda* and *Unani* of previous years was challenged in a troubled social and political atmosphere when differences between their practitioners became intense. General disbelief prevailed. *Hakims* denied the medical authority of the *vaids*.[76]

While integrating the two medical systems on a sound critical examination and scientific analysis, was the most viable solution to regaining the client base, a leading *vaidya*, P.S. Varier (1869–1958) and *Hakim* Ajmal Khan were satisfied with local princes and other rich elites as their chief patrons, who werenough to promote and bring them encomiums. On a different note, concerted efforts were made by the elites to further their relationship with the British style of life, made possible through two major institutions supported entirely by the local population. These were represented by the College of Fort William and Hindu College (later renamed, Presidency College).

Indigenous Collaboration: College of Fort William and Hindu College as Institutions for 'Proximity' with the British

The pivot of social and cultural change in imperial India may be viewed through Malinowski's[77] analysis of cultural institutions. According to Malinowski, "the invention of a new principle or technological device remains irrelevant unless studied in a cultural context and within a framework of organized activities." For him, an institution is 'the real isolate of cultural analysis.'[78] By this definition, the College of Fort William and Hindu College can be seen as prime institutions affording an analysis of Indian culture. The College of Fort William and Marquess Wellesley's 'Oxford of the East,' was set up in 1800 to train British civil employees. It was "the first European-created institution of higher learning in India to welcome Indians as faculty members and to encourage cultural exchange between Europeans and South Asians."[79]

The College of Fort William was not only an educational and training institution but a place which saw British-Indian interaction as a step toward the Orientalist rediscovery of Hindu classical and golden age. During the first three decades of nineteenth century, the Indian elites and educated intelligentsia, were a 'confused but optimistic individual striving to reconcile partially digested alien traits and unsatisfactory indigenous tradition.'[80] And almost a century later, they became the main supporters of Western medicine. The establishment of Hindu College on 27 August 1816 by the Calcutta *nouveaux riches* was an expression of the felt need to "provide the sons of that group with an advantageous European education."[81]

The establishment of the College of Fort William largely remained an extension of Hastings' policy which dictated that Indian cultural institutions should be retained as far as possible in order to establish a link between the 'ruler' and the 'ruled.' The College started as an Orientalist training centre, and for cultural and literary revival of Hindu learning, stems from Hastings' proficiency in Bengali, Urdu and Persian, and his belief that "the quickest route to the heart of a people is through the language of the country."[82]

Hastings' consistent policy and desire to understand Hindu culture and philosophy were continued by Wellesley in later years. It was through this institution that Wellesley was inclined to creating a class of Orientalised elites who were competent in their knowledge of classical culture and tradition. It was also premised on his belief that the institution would provide great benefits and best security to the public service in India. It is difficult to ascertain the motivation of Orientalists to train themselves in indigenous culture of the Hindus, although one thing can be said for certain. There was an element of interest in becoming masters of a new language and culture, or how else could Oriental enthusiasts, such as William Jones (1746–94), leave us a legacy of institutionalized learning; William Jones apparently was the first Englishman in India to visualize and establish a permanent institution of Oriental studies and research. The institution, called the *Asiatic Society* was established in 1784 with the aim of fulfilling William Jones' 'Asian dream' of learning the history, law, sciences, art, literature, and practically the entire knowledge of the Hindus. Besides, Jones' rediscovery of Sanskrit as the source of all languages of Indo-Europeans made him a seminal figure in the Orientalist search for India's rich heritage. As the foremost research institution, the *Society* led to the formation of major scientific and educational institutions in British India; the University of Calcutta (1857), and the Indian Science Congress (1913)[83] were fine examples of these changes. These developments also suggest an early interaction of Indian and Western intellectualism, by merging identities and interests of European colonialism and India.

The other institution that encouraged the process of acculturation and the exchange of cultural ideas was Hindu College. From its inception, Hindu College, 'the first collegiate institution of its kind anywhere in the West,'[84] was under the control of the few and new Calcutta elite, namely, P.K. Tagore, Radhakant Deb, and Ram Comul Sen. They had acquired much of their wealth through their long association with their British counterparts which facilitated and strengthened their appreciation of European culture, language and training. This also explains why the elitist patrons insisted on promoting European literature and sciences through the institution. It might seem that the College was founded with the aim of imparting secular knowledge in Western garb. Available evidence proves the contrary. The curriculum included, amongst other subjects, a detailed study of sacred Hindu law and grammar. Medical classes at the College focused on medicine and specialized courses on anatomy. Remnants of religious prejudice were still lingering when students performed major dissections on animals, at the same time were adept at handling human skeleton.

Practice of medicine at Hindu College changed notably with the establishment in 1831 of a hospital attached to the College where Hindu students could perform minor operations on human body. Although no Hindu had performed a major operation, they were recognized for their performance in minor operations.[85] Western medicine gradually gained acceptance with the expansion of medical education in the year 1831. A new hospital was founded at College to meet the increasing acceptance of Western medicine by that section of the Indian population who could afford the costs of Western education. Company rule and later, colonial rule, thus, became a history of contact of two civilizations, and of extensive networks of interaction, and of the unique processes of cultural exchange.[86] Within this arena of contact came other groups of people who, through previous associations with the British, became the main source of support to Western medical sciences. The following discussion will focus on how the urban elites in the erstwhile British Presidencies of Bombay and Bengal identified themselves with the British, became patrons of Western medicine, yet retained their traditional past only to join the nationalist struggle in later years.

A new chapter in the development of an intellectual tradition opened up at Hindu College with the appointment of Henry Louis Vivian Derozio (1809–31) as an instructor of English literature. His brief tenure from 1828 to 1831 ended with his untimely death due to cholera at age 22 in 1831. During this period, Derozio produced a minority of intellectuals who sought to reject Indian culture and identified themselves with the Western ideals. The group called *Young Bengal*, included high-caste Hindus, "usually one generation removed from the village and nurtured in Calcutta joint families surrounded by tightly-knit Bengali neighbors."[87]

If an overwhelming majority of Indian intellectuals in nineteenth-century Bengal identified themselves with India's past history, then how do we explain the origin of *Young Bengal* who had such a candid admiration for the West? The fact remains that *Young Bengal* was, by this time, already familiar with English learning at the modernizing and reforming traditional *patsalas*,[88] and was, for the first time, exposed to 'Macaulay-type' polarity between the superior West and their own tradition at Hindu College. Thus, while most of *Young Bengal* was ridiculing Hindu culture in the 1820s, one Kashi Prasad Ghose, disturbed by

Mill's indictment of Hindu polity in his *History of British India*, vehemently attacked and condemned Mill at the College examination; Ghose is the first known Bengali intellectual to openly defend Hindu identity despite his Western training.[89]

Parsis and *Bhadralok*: Indigenous Patrons of Western Medicine

In the preceding chapter we discussed how the Muslim royalty supported the art and practice of medicine amongst *Ayurvedic* and *Unani* physicians. This section will throw light on the continuity of success of *Parsis* as a social group during the rule of the British in terms of trade, commerce, industry as well as medicine. The *Parsi* clientele of Western medicine was, in fact, the early patrons of *Ayurveda* and *Unani* in medieval times. A brief sketch on the historical past of their settlements will allude to their gradual involvement in medical matters as part of their establishments in India.

The earliest settlements of *Parsis* in India were around 716 and 936 AD, when they were granted asylum by a Hindu king, Jadi Rana. As a kind gesture, and impressed by the *Parsi* priest who pledged his word, "we shall be the friends of India,[90] Jadi Rana assigned them a piece of land. The settlement was named Sanjan by the initial *Parsi* settlers. The name perhaps owes its origins to the city of Sanjan in Khorasan region of ancient Iran. It was from here that the early *Parsi* community made its way into the Western State of Gujarat.

In Gujarat, two regions known for the medical activities of *Parsis* were Surat and Navsari. It was here that around the sixteenth century, members of *Mehervaid* family began to be identified as hereditary medical practitioners, practicing Indian medicine for generations.[91] Thereafter, *Parsis* became interested in *Unani* medicine, and later as chief patrons of Western medicine.

As patrons of medical sciences under Muslim and colonial India, *Parsis* were also identified as successful medical practitioners. They were skilled in bone-setting, and as hereditary bone-setters, were called *Hadvaid* 'bone-physician, bone-setter.'[92] One such family of successful bone-setters was the Suralivala family from Madhi near Surat, where free services were offered to the local population, either in their clinics or patients' homes. In colonial India, the success of *Parsis* as a social group in the Indian society was partly attributed to the commercial expansion of Bombay in preceding years, and which ceded to the British in 1668; thereafter, it became an important area of interest for the British. By this time, the Mughal rule declined, thus paving the way for entry of the British into areas formerly supported by the Mughal royalty. Surat and Navsari regions of Gujarat were amongst these regions. As successful business magnates, *Parsi* traders gradually moved to the newly acquired the commercial city of Bombay, and became the first community to develop alliance with the British. The geographical mobility of *Parsis* had significant repercussions on their relation with the British, for it strengthened their social ties and opened up newer channels of trading with foreign lands in collaboration with the British. When the British made their way into Western India and China markets, *Parsis* supported them in expanding their business with China. With the passage of time, *Parsis,* "owing to their tradition of maritime trading, and their close connections with the British, shared in the profits of international trade."[93] This gave the *Parsis* of Bombay the much acclaimed higher status in comparison with *Parsis* in Surat and Navsari. It also earned them a substantial share in exporting cotton to Britain associated with the benefits of importing British textiles so that over a period of time, *Parsis* became the first traders to cherish the benefits of manufacturing indigenous cotton locally in Bombay.

> The *Parsis,* wrote William Milburn in 1813, rank next to the Europeans. They are active, industrious, clever, and possess considerable local knowledge. Many of them are very opulent, and each of the European houses of agency has one of the principal Parsee merchants concerned with it in most of their foreign speculations. They have become the brokers and banians (traders) of the Europeans. The factors belonging to these different houses in China, Bengal....are generally Parsees, and the correspondence is carried on in the country language, so that the British merchant knows no more than they communicate to him.[94]

In the field of medicine in colonial India, specifically during the eighteenth and early nineteenth centuries, families of *Parsi* practitioners were regarded highly for their ardent support for Western medical science. Most famous of these were Pestanji Ratanji Tamna (1757-1822), Kavasji Ratanji Tamna (1761-1818) and Behramji Bhikha, Sohrabji Jamshedji Doctor (1791-1852). Some *Parsis* were employed by the Company as a result of their close association with the British. Sohrabji Jamshedji Doctor joined the military hospital in 1819 keeping his private practice in later years in Surat. [95]

As close associates of the British, the *Parsis* benefited from them not only economically as industrial magnates, but also in terms of patrons of European sciences as pupils and as financial supporters. Thus, in 1830, Sir Jamshedji Jejeebhoy, first baronet, made a generous contribution to support a small charitable dispensary opened by Dr. Mackie, the first private practitioner who had established himself in the city in 1830. When Mountstuart Elphinstone retired as Governor of Bombay, a college of education in European sciences and literature was founded by the generous financial support from the *Parsis,* in honor of recognition of Elphintone's services. And when opportunities for medical education were opened up in Bombay, *Parsis* were the first one to take advantage of it. Sir Jamshedji Jejeebhoy later supported medical research at the Grant Medical College founded in 1845. Others joined his efforts by promoting various scientific and literary societies to encourage research not only in medicine but in other sciences. The first *Parsi* to join the College was Fardunji Jamshedji, and the first to receive a medical diploma from the college in 1851 was Meherwanji Sorabji Kharas. By 1884, amongst the several *Parsis* who qualified as physicians and surgeons, about 14 entered the lucrative Indian Medical Service through competitive examinations in London; some of them were appointed in higher positions in medical institutions. Dhanjisha Narozji Parakh, for instance, was appointed to the professorial Chair of midwifery at the Grant Medical College, and to the post of surgeon to the obstetric wad of the Sir Jamshedji Jijibhai (or Jejeebhoy) hospital.

With the growing popularity of Western medical sciences, the medical interests of *Parsis* expanded to incorporate the scientific essentials of indigenous medicine, with the added support of local princes. And the usual way of expressing allegiance was to dedicate their compilations to the royalty which also facilitated popular acceptance. In 1887, Rustomjee Naserwanjee Khory, Honorary physician at the Sir Jamshedji Jeejeebhoy Hospital, published 'The Bombay *Materia Medica* and Their Therapeutics,' expressing royal allegiance to promote and gain popular acceptance of the benefits of the *materia medica*. Here is how the book was dedicated :

The above author dedicates this book

To

His Highness

The Maharaja Sayajirao, Gaekawar of Baroda

Sena Khaskhel, Shamshere Bahadur,

As a Token of Admiration For

Many princely qualities and

As a humble tribute of gratitude

For

The zeal displayed in promoting the cause of

Native medical science in India

This work is

humbly dedicated

By

the Author[96]

In addition to Bombay as a city of successful *Parsis*, Bengal was marked by equally successful elite group called the *bhadralok* (or the 'high' and respectable people), identified by their unique sense of cultural values and social prestige. In effect, throughout the twentieth century colonial India, they remained a highly privileged and superior group,

> economically dependent upon landed rents and professional and clerical employment, keeping its distance from the masses by its acceptance of high-caste prescriptions and its command of education, sharing a pride in its language, its literate culture, and its history, and maintaining its communal integration through a fairly complex institutional structure that it had proved remarkably ready to adapt and augment to extend its social power and political opportunities.[97]

The *bhadralok* were mainly drawn from the three upper castes of Bengal, *Brahmin, Baidya* and *Kayastha*. The origin of *bhadralok* goes back to the late eighteenth century when high-caste Bengalis showed alacrity in investing in parts of land in response to new policies of land revenue. And by the nineteenth century, the Hindu and Muslim aristrocratic groups were replaced by the Hindu *bhadralok* who were happy with the idea of new possessions, for they became the landed class in colonial India. Because of the inordinate costs involved in Western and English education, sons of the landed *bhadralok* could benefit most from their association with the British. As British rule expanded, with an expansion in trade, military services, and more opportunities for Western-style education were opened up, the need to recruit local people became intense. In Bengal, the section of the population best placed to take advantage of the new appeal of Western medicine was the *bhadralok.*[98] Their support to English education gave paved their entry into the British professional and administrative services.

Although the basic distinction between *bhadra* and *abhadra*, or between the high and low, stemmed from the former's abstention from manual labor and their belief in the inferiority of manual occupations, medical practice remain unaffected by these prejudices. Western education almost became a hallmark of *bhadralok* status in colonial India, so that by the end of the nineteenth and early twentieth centuries, members of this group sought for their children

> education at the Presidency College, an English university or the Inns of Court in London, and success in the Indian Civil Service (I.C.S.) examination, at the Bar of the Calcutta High Court, or in one of the other learned professions of the capital. The school recorded in a Bengal government report in 1928, was the one gate to the society of the bhadralok.[99]

The Hindus in Bengal, and *Parsis* in Bombay were, thus, among the first to benefit from British trading and commercial activities. They were also the first to benefit from the capitalist enterprise which transferred from Britain to India in the early nineteenth century. The commercial interests of the British, successful as they were in creating a mercantile community in India, then depended on the cooperation of the middle classes for their expansion. *Parsis* and *bhadralok* provided the required support.

While the British private enterprise opened up new trade avenues in India, it also led to a rapid decline of indigenous industries, aggravated by an increasse in the imports of cotton goods. Nevertheless, *Parsis* were quick in responding to British call for industrial expansion, especially after 1813 when the general decline of Indian industries transferred industrial expansion to private traders. Not surprisingly, similarity in interests between the new middle classes and the British mercantile community often led the British in ranking *Parsis* as next to the Europeans.

Indigenous Medicine: Its Dwindling Clientele

The much written about religious prejudice did not stop the Indian clientele from moving over from *Ayurveda* and *Unani*, once the benefits of Western medicine were known and popularized, and even made accessible by Western practitioners. The fall in grace was a result of the loss of elites, and social classes who moved away from indigenous medicine. This was the most crushing blow to indigenous medicine[100] which did more harm to it than all the aspersions cast on it by the British. Western medicine was, for a long time, was for the British only. Around the early years of the twentieth century, however, the clientele of *Ayurveda* and *Unani* began to dwindle when the non-elite Indians got a taste of Western medicine in the moves made by colonial authorities to control epidemics like malaria,[101] and with the gradual production of Western-trained Indian doctors who set up this practice. The development of hospitals by the British from late nineteenth century onwards in various parts of the country, but mainly in metropolitan centers,[102] also made Western medicine more accessible to the local population, and the indigenous clientele, very slowly at first, began moving to Western medicine.[103]

Although Indian and Western forms of medical training were separated in 1835, the British continued their links through indigenous drugs. William Shaugnessy's *Bengal Pharmacopoeia*[104] was the first medical compendium based on indigenous drugs for medical practice in Bengal. Despite continued interest in Indian medicine, Western medicine moved away from indigenous medicine as a result of the increasing professionalization of medical knowledge, when medical practitioners discarded the humoral basis of Indian medicine and regarded indigenous medical knowledge as 'necessarily inferior.'[105] During the brief period of its existence, and by 1835, the *NMI* had already trained a new clientele of medical patrons in the form of *Native Doctors*. Its abolition, however, created an unanticipated void in the provision of medical services which was filled in by creating a class of Sub-Assistant Surgeons at the newly founded Calcutta Medical College. Thus, a secondary or military class was instituted where medical instructions were carried out in Indian vernaculars.

If we were to view colonial medical policies as part of colonial hegemony, and Western medicine as a 'tool of empire,'[106] then colonial moves in training local people, may well support this view. Besides, the demise of the *NMI* did it all. More students were trained for the European subordinate medical department, more classes were started in vernaculars which were developed into separate medical schools in the late nineteenth century; the Campbell Medical School founded in 1875 was one such example.

It is a truism that the British medical policy was never wholly focused on encouraging *Ayurveda* and *Unani* and in doing so, imperialist hubris may have played a critical role. It is also a truism that the superiority of British or Western-borne medicine in anatomical and surgical studies prompted the administrators to discontinue support to indigenous knowledge. The late nineteenth and early twentieth centuries witnessed new conflicts when indigenous practitioners defended indigenous medical science as 'science.' On the other hand, there was no move to ban *Ayurveda* by proscribing indigenously set up institutions. The 'stagnation' of indigenous medicine, perhaps, became evident at this stage of colonial rule. The British move to end classes at the *NMI*, and to introduce English as the language in the country paved the way for urban intelligentsia to voice their demands to preserve India's past. The Indian national movement was the result of this voice.

In Defense of Medicine: Medical Revivalism and the Indian National Movement

Nationalism in India was a political movement based on 'mingling of old ideas with new'[107] against the British administration. Never before, despite centuries of rule of the Muslims, did India visualize a concept of nationalism; the phenomenon was virtually absent until the spread of pervasive Western ideas through Western education, and Christianity under the British rule, made it difficult for India to evade the new ideological invasion. The anti-imperialist movement, thus, was a gradual outcome of this concern and the contradictions between the colonial imperatives and the different interests of the Indian population;[108] the movement embraced different classes and groups in India.[109]

The British in trying to supplant indigenous tradition and culture with the culture of the West, and presenting the west to the east, produced a cultural hybrid of all sorts. The presentation was from one small elite to another.[110] Spread of English education was the medium through which these measure were rendered complete. From the Indian side, the usual way of expressing resentment of Western ideas and way of life was sometimes through 'hitting back with their brains and pens,' as done by prominent members of Bengali elites, Rabindranath Tagore and Romesh Dutt.[111] In later years, however, the same group of people, as the most prominent and Western-educated group, united with the local population against British rule. The character of nationalism in India was, thus, shaped by a multitude of factors with an underlying feeling of discontentment with the British. Admittedly, the urban middle class was discontent with the high taxes, the increasing restrictions imposed on the educated Indians for entry into the British civil services, and with the disparity in salaries and offering benefits. In this context, nationalism represented an organized resistance to the colonial rule in India, organized on the firm belief and idea of 'India of national self-determination.'[112] In effect, Indian response to colonialism appeared to be twofold: one was nationalistic and revolutionary, and the other was Western and non-revolutionary. Nationalistic response expressed itself in various forms of cultural, religious and medical revival, with medical revivalism as part of appreciation of indigenous culture. The Western and non-revolutionary response, on the other hand, was expressed by the urban, educated middle class intelligentsia, represented by the *bhadralok* of Bengal, and the *Parsis* of Bombay.

In the mid-nineteenth century, members of the urban educated class became exponents of Hindu cultural nationalism who assumed that the degeneration of India and the destruction of its nationality were enhanced by the inroads that Western civilization had wrought upon the pristine heritage of India. By the mid-nineteenth century, however, nationalists included the same body of English-and Western-educated Indians. Although they comprised only a fraction of the total population, they dominated all professions including medicine, law and teaching. Nationalistic pursuits were also evident in the Presidency of Bengal which became the 'epicenter of the earthquake of Western ideas.'[113]

The partition of Bengal in 1905 intensified the nationalistic fervor, and expanded the scope of the movement making it a weapon of India's aspirations for political independence. Rabindranath Tagore, Bipin Chandra Pal, and Aurobindo Ghose were at the helm of the national movement expressions in Bengal. Not surprisingly, in the aftermath of the partition, all classes of people joined the national movement, and unanimously decided to boycott all foreign goods. Thus, the Landlords Association discouraged the merchant class from their dealings in Manchester cloth. Brahman priests announced their decision to curtail religious rites for those who would support foreign goods. It is known that professional men including doctors, lawyers, and teachers used their professional virtues to draw more people into the movement; they declared that they would not perform their services to those who expressed their unwillingness to participate. Religious institutions, the *Kali* temples for instance, were chosen as venues to take a pledge for defending the national identity, and to refrain from purchasing foreign goods.[114]

The move to revive India's culture and medical traditions also formed part of the movement. And since medical knowledge of the ancient Hindus was linked with the culture of the past, the move to resuscitate *Ayurveda* may be seen as a part of the rising national consciousness among the Indians. The movement accorded a prominent place to the revival of Sanskrit language and literature. The latter was said to represent the perennial fount from which the vernaculars of India were derived.[115] In fact, one of the basic assumptions of Hindu cultural nationalism was the belief that Hindu population constituted a religious and racial unity and the *Vedas*, which were believed to be the outgrowth of the Aryan intellect, were superior to anything the world had previously known.[116] Constant efforts were then made to popularize India's heritage to vindicate the superiority of indigenous culture and tradition against the much-vaunted capitalistic civilization of Europe.[117] The feeling of cultural nationalism was so intense that the national movement was often considered synonymous with it.[118] Alongside the revivalist efforts of *Ayurveda*, those of *Unani* medicine also came to the fore at the height of the national movement. The Muslim community began to identify the vicissitudes of Muslim cultural past, believing in revitalizing the glory of Muslim culture, at the same time working with an open attitude of 'improving' medical science. One name that is often associated with regeneration of indigenous medical science as a cultural symbol that of Musihul-Mulk *Hakim* Mohammed Ajmal Khan (1868–1927). Coming from a family of renowned physicians of Sharif Khani family who served the Mughal courts and local princes in British India, Ajmal Khan devoted himself to promoting a systemized version of medical knowledge. His efforts were best seen in producing literary writings to reach the people—an exhaustive manual on the plague epidemic in 1897, and a medical journal, *Mujalla-i-Tibbia* in 1901–02, exemplify his literary achievements. As the most influential Muslim political leader, he was considered "the nearest the Muslims had to Gandhi in terms of breadth of political appeal: he was highly regarded by government, respected in the Congress, and amongst Hindus generally, and was one of the few Muslims who could feel equally at home among *ulama, nawabs* and (Westernized) Aligarh graduates."[119]

Descendants of *hakims,* who practiced in the courts of Mughal regime prior to the British, were faced with intense political situations that prompted the cause of Indian nationalism even further. This happened when special grants in the forms of *jagir*, assigned to successful medical practitioners by the Muslim royalty in recognition of their services, were taken over by the British as they took over a particular area. Records show that a family of *hakims* in Kalanaur (Punjab) and a family of *vaids* in Amritsar in the northwest part of India lost their *jagir*, and hence a prosperous medical school was reduced to an institution with only a handful of students left during British rule.[120] With the growing cultural, and later economic and political nationalism in the country, *Unani* medicine was made part of the Muslim political symbols. The foundations of the movement also lay in the popular belief that British rule became the major cause of India's economic backwardness. The Indian population, recognizing that imperialism was a barrier to the general development, felt and bewailed the economic exploitation of the country.[121] The destruction of traditional industries led to a progressive impoverishment of the peasant. The policy of exacting the largest possible land-revenue led to a great devastation which was made worse by the meager economic returns peasants received in exchange. Very little was spent on agriculture, and a very large sum was spent on meeting the needs of the British administration serving the interests of British trade and industry. Bholanath Chandra and Chandra Nath Bose were among the prominent advocates of economic nationalism, striving assiduously for the subversion of British policy.[122] In addition to the economic and cultural nationalist doctrines, the nationalistic Indians espoused a doctrine of political nationalism, the great consummating point of union of which was premised on the fact that 'as subjects of the same foreign, all Indians enjoyed common rights and privileges.'[123] Political nationalism, thus, laid down the necessity of securing power of control over provincial affairs. Even for medical revival, efforts towards educational and institutional changes were an outgrowth of the rising political nationalism. An important change in education during this period was respresented by the foundation of the *Unani* Medical School for Women by *Hakim* Ajmal Khan in 1908, and years later, liberal education in supporting the establishment of Jamia Millia Islamia University in Delhi became his aim. In 1921, he established the *Ayurvedic* and *Unani Tibbia* College where *Ayurvedic* and *Unani* medical sciences formed the core curriculum alongwith courses in Western medicine. Following his death, The Institute of History of Medicine and Medical Research in Tughlaqabad, continued extensive research activities on the Indian pharmacopoeia utilizing the scientific methods of Western medicine.With a mission for resuscitating India's medical heritage, his association with Mahatma Gandhi earned him a political and national fame for Hindu-Muslim unity identified by common interests in indigenous medical knowledge. Suffice it to say that these changes took place through a series of professionalizing processes of 'resecularizing' medical systems—in terms of changing from scientific medicine to religious forms, and after independence re-formulated as scientific.[124] Although medical practice ranged from belief in the scientific principles of *Unani* medicine to belief in God as the ultimate healer of all diseases, there were repeated attempts at recognizing the merits of the Western sciences as well as maintainng the popular appeal of indigenous medicine.

The introduction and spread of English as the medium of instruction in all disciplines throughout the country also intensified the national movement. English was not only declared as the official language, but also became the medium through which the knowledge of English literature was sought to be disseminated, aided by the printing press. Those interested in receiving English education were disappointed by imperial dictates that mass-education in English was impracticable because of the limited funds ear-marked for educational purposes. The result was that only a fraction of the population could afford English education to facilitate easy interaction between the imperial administrators and the indigenous population; the expansion of commercial activity in the Presidency of Bengal called for further expansion of English education, albeit to a small section of the population. Cultural nationalism, an outgrowth of the conflict between the local population and the rulers, was further precipitated by the need to establish a Western value system of education among the people whose customs and traditions were profoundly different those from those of the former. The situation, when applied to the revivalism of indigenous traditions, bears different results. McCully[125] argument that the feeling of national unity was inculcated among the Western-educated Indians alone is debtable. For we know that several *Ayurvedic* enthusiasts were not part of the English education stream, yet dominated all discussions and remained at the helm in their fight against colonialism.

The recognition that contemporary traditional practices do not reflect the significant achievements of the ancient civilization as a result of their decline, due largely to the impositions of an alien culture, and the subsequent demand for State patronage or governmental interference from new regimes for their resuscitation, figure as important features of most revivalist movements in South-Asian history.[126] This, proposition is, however, disputable. The alien nature of British rule cannot be held responsible for lack of progress in Indian medicine. Under Muslim rule in India, it was seen that although the kings, princes and rulers did not share the same cultural heritage they ruled, they did not neglect *Ayurveda* and, on the contrary, extended common patronage to *Ayurvedic* and *Unani* practitioners at the royal courts. So what was it in Western medicine that made it look so different from the traditional forms of medicine? We must realize that Western medicine, at least in the twentieth century, was an offshoot of paradigmatic work when its practitioners were engaged in solving scientific puzzles, to use Kuhn's[127] notion of scientific paradigms. By comparison, Western medicine expressed itself as a different form which made Indian medicine seem stagnant and in a state of comatose. By this definition, imperialist hauteur may have had a role to play in bringing Indian medicine to this state, although one might also argue that this was a sequel to the marked internal differences germane in both. After all, the early period of British rule in India coincided with the period of medical reform in Britain in the second half of eighteenth and middle of the nineteenth century.

The feeling of lack of development in *Ayurveda*, thus, was accentuated and became evident with the proliferating advances in the West. This provided a further spur in the nationalistic efforts to revive Indian medicine and to bring it on par with its Western counterpart, and closely identified by its proponents as essential for revitalizing the 'glory of the past.' Some of them actively took the cause of Indian medical science as part of the religious reform movement in mid-nineteenth century. The foremost revivalist was Dayanand Saraswati, a Gujarati Brahman (1824–1883), founder of the most powerful Hindu reform organization, the *Arya Samaj* (Society of the Aryans). Dayanand Saraswati's rejection of the superiority of the West inspired Hindus to unite on the basis of *Vedic* religion. Since ancient medical science in India had *Vedic* origins, it was considered superior to any progress in the West. His reason for restoring Hinduism and ancient science and wisdom was more in his passion and respect for Indian knowledge than in disbelief for Western ideas. For he saw every scientific and medical discovery in the West as an outcome of the knowledge contained in the *Vedas*, arguing that "the science of the West was but the realization of the scientific programme anticipated by the seers of the East thousands of years ago."[128] Nationalist interpretations of Indian culture at this point also drew from growing propensities towards establishing an Indian identity and the superiority of the past.

Conforming to the idealized traditions, the nineteenth-century reformers engaged themselves in revivifying Indian culture. The political and social reforms made by the colonial administrators, also created awareness amongst the Muslim population which linked the decline of Muslim society and culture to colonial rule, although in reality they were held responsible for the spiritual and moral decadence. Conformity to traditions by Muslim society was the most obvious outcome of this. Alongside, Islamic movements, Hindu reform movements also characterized late nineteenth-century dynamism as a result of colonial penetration. Contrary to etablishing a degree of standardization of cultural traditions, some indigenous practitioners became part of a group that questioned the efficacy of medical science. At a time when anti-imperialist feelings were heightened at all levels of Indian society, fresh interpretations of Indian traditions reigned supreme among Indian intellectuals and Hindu and Muslim nationalists. Thus, in 1878, *Hakim* Afdal Ali, in his *Jamiush-Shifaiya*, challenged the theories of Greek medicine, while *Hakim* Abdul Majid (1883–1922), a *Unani* physician of repute, founded a clinic and a pharmacy shop, *Hamdard*, in Delhi in 1906. As the name suggested, 'sharing the pain of others,' the clinic became popular amongst the local people. Few years later, he converted the small clinic into a pharmacy manufacturing and selling indigenous drugs all throughout the country; it was called *Hamdard Dawakhana.*[129] Successful as it was over the years, it was taken over by *Hakim* Majid's youngest son, Mohammad Said, who established branches of *Hamdard* in Pakistan after its creation in 1947.

The movement to revive *Ayurveda* proved to be one of major significance in Indian history, and aimed at achieving recognition and status by seeking State patronage and establishing institutions. The movement found expression in 1907 with the establishment of the All India *Ayurvedic Mahasammelan* (All India *Ayurvedic* Conference) which coincided with the popularity of *Hakim* Ajmal Khan as the political leader and supporter of *hakims*. At the seventh session of the All India Ayurvedic Mahasammelan, held in Madras, the rich armamentarium and their medicinal value in *Ayurvedic* practice were emphasized. In his Presidential address,[130] *Kaviraj* Jaminibhushan Ray, Fellow of Calcutta University, stated that "there was plenty of room for a systematic study and investigation of medicinal plants in *Ayurveda*. This will be done by providing facilities in the form of establishing colleges and hospitals, and gardens for a study of medicinal plants." This followed a remark made by the then Emperor, George V: "you have to conserve the ancient learning and simultaneously to push forward Western science."

Although, in the 1850s and 1860s, the British employed *Unani* practitioners as part of extending medical relief to the local population, they denied them official status during the early part of twentieth century. The real blow then came between 1912 and 1919 when Western and Indian practitioners trained in Western medicine 'de-professionalized' the practice of indigenous medicine by prohibiting indigenous physicians from participating in any legal dispute or providing medical certificate for illness to workers. This was expressed through the various Registration Acts passed between 1912 and 1919 in the Presidencies of Madras, Bombay and Bengal, and in the United Provinces, Burma, Bihar and Orissa, and by a Medical Degrees Act which restricted the use of the title of 'Doctor.'[131] This was a sequel to the establishment of the All India *Ayurvedic* Congress in 1907, as part of the *Ayurvedic* revivalist efforts; most members of the Congress, which was entirely voluntary, were leading practitioners of indigenous medicine. The movement was, perhaps, seen as a threat and a major step towards achieving medical monopoly, also evident from repeated pleas by indigenous practitioners for better government positions. The partition of Bengal in 1905 into Hindu Bengal and Muslim Bengal, based on the religion of the majority, intensified this move. It left the people of India with total distrust in British intentions. In the meanwhile, British and Indian physicians (trained in Western medicine) received constant threats of expulsion and de-registration from medical officers in Britian, for violating the British ethical codes of medicine by associating with their indigenous counterparts.[132] This intensified anti-British feelings in the country. Economic deprivation as a result of limited white-collar employment compounded with population increase in the late nineteenth and early twentieth centuries exacerbated a disbelief in colonial administration. At the same time, and during the War years, the British administrators sought to improve the existing medical techniques after a communication from the then Director-General of the Indian Medical Services, Sir Pardey Lukis, in 1916 where he declared that "the improvement of the training of *hakims* and *vaids* is a part of the present policy of Government because for many years to come, they will constitute the medical attendants of by far the largest portion of the Indian community."[133]

In view of this recognition, the first integrated *Unani-Tibbiya* College was established in Delhi in 1916 where students received combined medical instructions in biomedical topics along with *Ayurveda* and *Unani*. Subsequent proposals for similar establishments were, however, turned down, when in 1918 *Hakim* Ajmal Khan was disappointed when the Imperial Legislative Assembly dismissed the possibility of 'placing the ancient and indigenous system on a scientific basis.'[134]

> The opinion unanimously expressed by local Government is that it is practically impossible to place the indigenous systems of medicine on a scientific basis. The systems are a survival of medical knowledge that once prevailed in Europe, but has been superseded by a series of scientific investigations and discoveries extending over several centuries. They ignore the instruments of scientific investigation that have been made modern medicine and surgery possible, and the theories on which they are based are demonstrably unsound.[135]

New concessions were embodied through the Montagu-Chelmsford Reforms of 1919 when the rights and responsibility for health provisions was transferred from the imperial to provincial government under Indian ministers. Indians then assumed a new role in governing the country from the time of World War I and the Reforms which increasingly linked the *Ayurvedic* movement with nationalist politics. The creation of a new system of *dyarchy*, or dual-government, in Indian provinces divided the administrative sector into 'reserved' and 'transferred' categories. In accordance with this, revenue, finance and law were treated as 'reserved' categories under the rule of the governors, while health, education and sanitation, and public health, amongst others, became 'transferred' subjects under the responsibility of the local ministers.[136] Gradually, the increasing entry of Indians into the legislature made it easier for nationalists and advocates of Indian medicine to voice their demands in favor of the regeneration of India's rich cultural heritage.

The transfer of responsibility did not imply a change in the British perception of indigenous medicine. As a result, continued hostility and disfavor were conspicuous in imperial policies and attitude, both of which found expression in their attempts to label Western or allopathic medicine as 'modern scientific medicine.'[137] While imperial policies attempted to keep the Indian society under control at the height of the nationalist agitation by giving some concessions through their reform policies, this did not stop the Indian nationalists and *Ayurvedic* revivalists from demanding equal recognition. In the 1920s, management of indigenous medicine was the stated goal of provincial governments. The Indian National Congress, as the leading voice of political and nationalist opinions on reforming cultural traditions in response to colonial rule, supported the revivalist movement by demanding State patronage for *Ayurveda*, and passed a resolution in favor of popularization of schools, colleges and hospitals of indigenous medicine. Not long after this, in 1921, Shyamadas Vacaspati, a reputed *Ayurvedic* scholar, founded a national university of Bengal, called *Gaudiya Saravidyayatana* which was later expanded to include an *Ayurvedic* Wing; the latter was established in the University to protest against the introduction of Western-oriented education of the day. In the same year, Mahatma Gandhi inaugurated another *Ayurvedic* College in Delhi followed by a hospital in Calcutta. In 1923, an *Ayurvedic* Committee was formed in Bengal to promote *Ayurvedic* learning through a central *Ayurvedic* College. The proposed College was the work of the sub-committee of the *Ayurvedic* Committee which suggested an amalgamation of the then existing three *Ayurvedic* Colleges—*Astanga Ayurvedic* College, *Baidyashastrapith* and the *Govinda Sundari Ayurvedic College*, into a central institution where both Indian and Western sciences could be taught. After several debates and exchange of proceedings between the Committees, the Secretary, the Board of Trustees and the Governing Body, the proposed College won the favor for the promotion of *Ayurvedic* learning.[138]

While *Ayurvedic* physicians adopted strategies in defense of the scientific basis of indigenous science, *hakims* also were quick to react to British views of Indian medicine, as stagnant. Liebeskind provides interesting arguments on how *hakims*, frustrated with the policies of the colonial establishment, proved its efficacy by arguing for *Unani-Tibb* as a systematic and scientific body of knowledge. Thus, reiterates Liebeskind, "*Unani-tibb* was accused of not being a medical 'system' of being wrong, dogmatic, old, inflexible; of being only popular because it was cheap and its clients ignorant."[139]

The defense of *Unani* as science owes much to the work of eminent *hakims* who came from influential families practicing *Unani* medicine for generations. *Hakim* Ajmal Khan, Kabir al Din, and Abd al Latifre made systematic attempts at not only proving its scientific basis but also made sure that they did this in the optic of Western medicine, or even re-interpreting the relevance of the textual traditions. They started their defense on the premise '*Unani tibb* was a science.'[140] At a time when political nationalists were seeking Muslim identity, Muhammad Iqbal (1873–1938), a renowned poet and philosopher, gave the Muslim intellectuals a new view for this identity; he also provided a framework for Pakistan.[141] The political changes in the early part of the twentieth century further aggravated the visibility of Hindus and Muslims as two different communities and identities resulting from religious nationalism.

The development of an *Ayurvedic* college at Poona illustrates the politicization of medical revival in the post-war period during which there were increasing problems of student unrest in *Ayurvedic* colleges. The Civil Disobedience or the Non-Cooperation Movement prodded students to boycott British-aided schools and foreign goods. They actively responded to the call and began to boycott universities throughout India, as part of the Non-Cooperation Campaign. At Poona, political leaders founded a university after the nationalist hero, Lokmanya Tilak, with *Ayurveda* as one of the courses of study. But in 1932, the institution was de-recognized and students of the University were imprisoned for participating in the second Civil-Disobedience Campaign of 1930-34, which was fought more intensely than previous efforts. As a reaction to this attitude, a new college of *Ayurveda* was founded by the leaders of the *Ayurvedic* movement in 1933 in Poona. By 1955, the College had gained State recognition and achieved affiliation to Poona University. It eventually became one of the best-equipped *Ayurvedic* colleges in the country. Notwithstanding such attempts, the movement met with partial success. Though it was successful in establishing a large number of educational institutions, it failed to set up uniform courses of training and professional opportunities for graduates in the field, with variations between States or even within the same region. Brass describes in some detail the reasons for the failure of the move to promote *Ayurveda*. One reason was the internal conflict among the revivalists on educational and professional standards.[142] Arguments between the two wings of the movement—one favoring reliance on ancient texts for promoting *shuddha* or *pure Ayurveda*, and the other advocating complete integration of the latter with modern medicine—resulted in formulating an *Ayurvedic* curriculum with unaccountable variations. The recognition that *pure Ayurveda* was unable to handle the public health needs of India led the advocates to frame a system of *Ayurvedic* education embodying concurrent instructions in Indian and Western medical sciences. This was specifically designed to train students in the fundamental aspects of *Ayurveda* while simultaneously imparting knowledge of Western medical science.[143] The shift to a focus on what was ideal in medical practice was a result of the pressure from the urban, Western-educated indigenous elites who viewed indigenous medicine as 'stagnant' against the so-called scientific dynamism in Western medicine. Integrating the two seemed the most viable option for taking care of public health demands. But a common understanding on the feasibility of an effective integration of the two systems of medicine because of the fundamental differences underlying the two, led the proponents of *pure Ayurveda* and leaders of the *Ayurvedic* Congress, to outright protest against such a move; instead, they demanded its immediate abolition and replacement by *shuddha Ayurvedic* studies.[144] Thus, differences over the curriculum and the innate dissimilarities with its Western counterpart influenced the way in which medical reform was perceived under the framework of political nationalism.

At the provincial level, the government adopted measures in the 1920s to support indigenous medicine by supervising its education through schools and colleges, and by regulating medical practice. This became more apparent at the turn of the twentieth century when the Imperial State was pushed into making definite decisions about the future of Indian medicine. It is possible that pressure from the national movement may have inspired changes in this direction. Provincial governments which were set up in the early twentieth century, and were continued in post-independent India, gave *Ayurveda* some measure of support during the period. Several State governments set up Boards of Indian medicine to look into the status of Indian medical science. In addition, each province had branches of the *Ayurvedic* Congress to present the needs and demands of indigenous practitioners before the provincial governments, as government institutions regulating indigenous practitioners. A government school of *Ayurveda* was then set up as early as 1887 and later, in 1908. A committee appointed by the Mysore government, viewing the lack of practical emphasis in *Ayurveda*, recommended fortification of education in traditional medicine with anatomy, physiology and surgery in the curriculum.[145] By this time, study of anatomy, physiology and surgery was considered important for the medical curriculum in the west, and recognizing the validity of scientific breakthroughs achieved by earlier men of science in the West, most Indians also believed that integrating the knowledge of the two systems would be the most optimum solution. Though institutions offering courses in *Ayurveda* and *Unani* proliferated, their setting was deemed inappropriate and 'dismal.' The *Tibbiya* College founded in Hyderabad in 1890, the Aryan Medical School founded in Bombay in 1896, and the Government *Ayurvedic* College of Mysore founded in 1905,[146] were amongst those condemned. They were seen as 'ill-equipped' without laboratories or libraries. Gradually, with more patronage of the princely states and caste and religious associations, additional schools and dispensaries began to emerge in different parts of the country so that by 1947, there were as many as 57 urban *Ayurvedic* and *Unani* schools with access to hospital wards for clinical instructions, laboratories and dissection halls. But despite such a positive improvement, the state of schools was what Leslie candidly remarked, "enough to expose the scandal of the ancient medical systems."[147] This may have been a sequel to the widening gap between indigenous medicine, seen as based on memorization of medical verses and 'cookbook' instructions for the preparation of medicinal drugs, and Western medicine with a dynamic base of medical diagnosis and treatment. In order to address the growing differences, the central government appointed a series of Committees in the Indian provinces to look into aspects of promoting, and regulating the development of indigenous systems of medicine. The Madras Committee (1921), for instance, realized that as body of science, Indian medicine was strictly scientific and logical, and had a willing clientele at the rural level. Lack of surgical and anatomical studies were not considered unimportant. And in order rectify this 'defect,' the government of Madras established a school of Indian medicine with the sole aim of imparting integrated education in indigenous and Western sciences. About the same time, the government of Bengal set up separate committees for *Ayurveda* and *Unani*. It was not until 1922 that the official plan for complete integration of indigenous and Western medicine was taken up by Usman Committee (1922), headed by Muhammad Usman who recognized that *Ayurveda* was based on viable and scientific theories but its practice had become deficient over the years. And in order to supplement this gap, the committee demanded an incorporation of the technology of modern medicine, particularly in surgery and diagnostics. Its recommendations were opposed by Western as well as traditional practitioners some of whom condemned *Ayurveda* as an 'obsolete' science while others saw the proposal as falling against the orthodox prejudices of contact with human bodies for anatomical practice. Notwithstanding opposition from Western medical professionals and advocates of *shuddha Ayurveda,* attempts in favor of founding new institutions with combined instructions in modern and Indian medicine continued.[148] After all, this was the first time an official attempt was made by a local government to subject indigenous medicine to scientific scrutiny. The outcome of further investigations were seen in the establishment of the School of Indian Medicine in Madras in 1924 where medical teaching included parallel instructions in *Ayurveda*, *Unani* and *Siddha (shuddha)* medicine.[149] The first Health Ministers' Conference held in 1946, gave a new dimension to Indian medicine when it passed a resolution pressing the need for more research in indigenous medicine, and for establishing new colleges and schools, recruiting Indian practitioners in the health services of the country.[150] The genesis of this resolution is found in the Bhore Committee, founded by Sir Joseph Bhore in 1946. The Committee's report, published in 1946, provided guidelines for health planning in the following fifteen years, but failed to account for the utility of indigenous medicine in the health services of the country, a move which was heavily criticized by *Ayurvedic* exponents, when members of the Committee argued that "no system of medical treatment which was static in conception and practice, and did not keep pace with the discoveries and researches of scientific workers of the world over, could hope to give the best available ministration to those who sought its aid."[151]

At the same time, the Committee acknowledged that the treatment given by practitioners of traditional medicine was cheap, and that the empirical knowledge accumulated over centuries, had resulted in a fund of experience which was of some value.[152] The final decision on utilizing indigenous medicine was, however, left to the provincial governments. Amidst a state of uncertainty and confusion about the future of Indian medicine, the Committee was successful in establishing a separate department of history of medicine at a teaching hospital and College in Delhi—the All India Institute of Medical Sciences—for research and study of indigenous systems with a view to finding out their scope in the medical relief; this revived a hope for State support to indigenous practitioners.[153]

The emphasis on concurrent teaching and integration of *Ayurvedic* and Western sciences was stressed by the Chopra Committee, headed by R. N. Chopra. In comparison with Western sciences, the Committee highlighted the scientific adequacy and technological deficiency of *Ayurveda* but also recommended its professionalization in combination with Western medicine.[154] The idea was to encourage scientific research in Indian medicine and achive a synthetic medical system with significant aspects of both.

Colonial India and Medicine: Concluding Reflections

From the foregoing discussion, few remarks can be made in conclusion. It is apparent that in colonial India, indigenous medicine was recognized as a viable and a better alternative for extending medical relief to the people. This meant that both had a large and willing clientele base which brought encomiums to its practitioners enabling them to amass huge fortunes. The relentless efforts of the indigenous population in reviving India's cultural heritage and the national movement incorporating Indian systems of medicine, gave further inspiration for indigenous medicine to re-establish its lost status. In addition, patronage to Indian medicine during colonial India was characterized by three groups. Included in these were the *Ayurvedic* enthusiasts, who were part of the Indian national movement and strove to revive medicine as part of India's Golden Age, the Provincial committees which were formed to promote and develop indigenous learning, in the best way possible either by strengthening its adequacies or by collaboration with the Western medical science; the view dominated all discussions in the first two decades of the twentieth century when the urban elites, the Western-educated Indians, and the nationalists made medical revival their favorite area of religious and cultural revitalization. Finally, indigenous practitioners also formed a willing support-base; they never welcomed the idea of their practice receding into the background by the inroads Western medicine had made either seen as a dynamic science or as a system fully supported by the State.

At this point it is logical to contend that in spite of political patronage to indigenous medicine in ancient and medieval periods, and later State support, Indian medicine was perhaps unable to pick up the same extent of dynamism exhibited by its Western counterpart. Perhaps, the biggest blow to Indian medicine was the movement of its established clientele to Western medicine. State sponsorship of Western sciences facilitated the move, making it easier to reach the local population, so that by the twentieth century proposals to integrate indigenous and Western medical traditions were seen as the best option for advancing the status of Indian medicine. The above contentions may lead one to believe that by the time British left India, indigenous medicine exhibited 'a less dynamic character' not on par with its Western counterpart. However, I take a different position with respect to this. The patrons of indigenous medicine, its practitioners, the enthusiastic nationalists, and the provincial patrons and local governments, all produced a cumulative effect on the medical profession during colonial India. Thus, judged by its scientific attributes, Indian medicine was fully dynamic and professional in its medical practice. The imperial administrators with their political dictates of hegemonic imperatives were unable to establish monopoly of Western medicine which existed as 'one amongst the many' medical systems flourishing in India. Both Indian and Western forms of medical traditions had an independent professional trajectory to follow, guided by total acceptance, accommodation or, at times, rejection of their counterpart. By the end of the colonial rule, thus, there were several competing medical systems, with no hierarchical or monopolizing attributes—quite akin to medical pluralism.

In addition, medical work in pre-colonial India consisted mainly of literary progress in medical science. Quite often these successes were the result of new discoveries and new therapeutic drugs for specific ailments which enriched the medical compendia produced at the time. Progress in this direction did not go well with the British when they gave indigenous learning a more empirical base. Thus, it seems that additions to the *Ayurvedic* lore did not help in revitalizing medical knowledge, which is why protests were made to take anither look and study Indian medical sciences with a Western outlook. The fact is that although medical knowledge was never lost through these accretions, the real spur in policy shifts came when Western medicine exposed the differences between the two systems of knowledge. Competition, struggle, accommodation, and survival of plural medical systems with a willing clientele base, were the the most conspicuous outcome of these distinctions.

Conclusions

Political Ideology and Medical Traditions in India

In drawing upon the interplay between medical thought and political, some major themes come to the fore. One theme that is consistent in this work is the role played by the ruling ideology in guiding the sphere of medical activities. In ancient times, this association started with medical encounters in which the 'intellectual curiosity' of medical men settled down to an unquestioning technology at the behest of the State. Peaceful as it all seemed, initially, when the same medical men questioned the scriptural declarations of the ruling religious ideology with an empirical focus, their practice faced *medical demise.* Although, a closer examination of various compilations of *Ayurveda* reveals that there was a conscious effort by physicians to avoid this fate by providing a mythological veneer to *brahmanize* medical knowledge, it made their scientific and medical observations 'unscientific.' At a later date, the rational period in India, from about 1000 B.C.E., produced some of the most fascinating series of debates on what constitutes the 'scientific method.' In reflecting upon the validity of the role of the State in determining the prospects of medical knowledge and practice, thus, it is evident that the State saw itself 'strategizing' medical affairs in anticipation of a possible threat to the teleological harmony on which religious theories and political beliefs rested. This was because knowledge of religious scriptures became less powerful in the presence of medical knowledge of *Ayurvedic* practitioners which provided an alternative framework of professional power. The questioning and challenging nature of medical science endangered its practice in relation to the political State. More conclusively, in line with this development, without undermining the significance of the State, it can be asserted that State patronage is not essential for the success of medicine as an art, but perhaps for medical practice, especially when its practitioners make calls to promote its validity.

Under Muslim rule in India, medicine became a 'syncretic' profession built upon the scientific essentials of *Ayurveda* and *Unani* medicine. In this period, we have challenged the popular belief of the decline of Indian medicine under the Muslim royalty. As such, there was no hostility between the two medical systems; at least our sources and interpretations indicate so. Hence, in the absence of any definite evidence which would suggest that *Ayurveda* or its practitioners were being persecuted, it may be concluded that Muslim rulers made elaborate and unabated attempts to coordinate the two medical traditions. These efforts were best seen in the proliferation of medical compendia and scrolls produced at the behest of the grand emperors. Quite often, the size of the medical compilation was a measure of its worth, and hence of the reputation of the author—the grander the compendia, the more enviable his position. Almost every physician aspired to win the confidence of the royalty, establishing a 'long-term bond' as a successful physician at the royal courts. The *Mughal* emperors, in particular, earned the reputation of being staunch supporters and generous patrons of art, learning and administrative talent. It is little surprising then that in the early Muslim settlements, and later in the Mughal period, several foreigners, majority of whom were either Afghans or Turans (Iranian) from Shiraz region of Iran, went to India to seek their fortune. They were mainly poets, lawyers, and physicians who found much favor with the ruling emperors at the time.

Although medical practitioners serving the royalty in their courts enjoyed greater social prestige and benefits of a royal association, those working with the various middle classes, especially the petty officials, the revenue officials, and the *mansabdars*, thrived equally well outside the royal environment which was also strengthened by Mughal policies of social integration of the middle classes into the imperial administration. This means that the success of a practical body of knowledge, such as medicine, is contingent not upon the political State but upon a dependable and willing clientele base or a 'medical market place' which would promote the flow of medical services. The prosperity of *hakims* and *vaids* was catalyzed by the Hindu and Muslim nobility under the Mughal rule which although

> suffered from a number of internal weaknesses, was on a broad view, a remarkable institution which welded into a homogenous and harmonious whole, men belonging to different regions and tribes, speaking different languages and professing different religions, and with differing cultural traditions. The *Mughals* succeeded in imbuing the nobles with a sense of common purpose and loyalty to the reigning dynasty, in imparting to them a distinctive cultural outlook, and in creating traditions of high efficiency and endeavor in administration. It was, thus, a definite factor in securing for a century and a half a remarkable degree of unity and good government in the country.[1]

Apart from the existence of an exclusive clientele for both *Ayurveda* and *Unani*, the common scientific paradigms of medical knowledge and practice, recognized in terms of identical governing assumptions of humoral theory and pharmacopoeia, also facilitated common patronage to the two medical traditions.

Professional and social mobility of medical professionals at various levels within the system made it possible for them to have sufficient mobility to move to a new and better social stratum in terms of earning a living. Ironically, movement of individuals from one geographical location to another synchronized with a change in their professions.[2] Such was the freedom of mobility under the emperors.

Kuhn's notion of scientific discoveries and paradigms to assess the relevance of the scientific discoveries made in pre-colonial India, would be worth a fresh look at this stage. Gauging by his approach to studying the 'act of discovery through an interpretation of the history of science,' it cannot be discounted that the work of earlier men of science in the form of medical compendia, were not mere accretion of discoveries; they reflected a scientific approach to medical inquiry, often recorded after several scientific trials. The following quote proves our contention. "Contrary to appearances, the growth of science is not a cumulative process but rather takes place through a series of revolutionary realignments of basic concepts. Each of these revolutions exhibits a similar general pattern in which the act of discovery emerges."[3] The content of the medical compilations, thus, has to be seen as constituting a pattern of scientific development which places a single discovery, be it of treatment practices by herbs, within this pattern and is subsequently explained with reference to a social context in which the act of discovery was made.

The discussion on medicine in the imperial rule revealed some provocative findings, made more interesting by the introduction of Western medicine. The period, thus, witnessed an interplay between the imperial imperatives and the plural medical systems represented by *Ayurveda*, *Unani* and their Western counterpart. Once again, in maintaining our position in defiance of the argument that indigenous medicine was denied all forms of support by the imperialists, we can argue that it was during the British rule that Indian medicine was for the first time seen as 'stagnant.' Rapid advances in technology, anatomy, surgery and allied sciences, provided measures against which Indian medicine was subject to medical scrutiny. For they led to different ways of viewing disease and health conditions, as agents justifying power and control. Added to this was the promotion of education in English, the limited benefits of which nurtured a new social group—the Western-educated Indian elite which "surfaced as modern subjects who could claim to represent and act upon the subaltern masses from whom they distinguished themselves,"[4] respresenting, what I would call, an *association-dissociation-association* identity complex in relation to Indian culture.

The readiness with which the British empire is blamed for the lack of appeal in Indian medicine is because for the first time the medical differences between the two became obvious. While colonial hegemony, monopoly and imperial power may have played a significant role in determining the beneficiaries of State and official patronage, they were legitimized, or at least seemed so, by the marked differences between Indian and Western medicine. This inspired the imperial administrators to acquire newer forms of control giving wide berth to its Indian counterpart, and hence disregard its scientific essentials during most part of the seventeenth and eighteenth centuries.

The second half of the nineteenth century and much of the twentieth century witnessed conflicting opinions on what constituted 'science.' In their defense of indigenous medicine as scientific, practitioners often wondered how an ever-changing content of medical knowledge in Western medicine could be called scientific. For them, "no progressive science could call itself perfect or complete without a re-interpretation of literary texts of earlier periods."[5] Much of the nineteenth century witnessed Indian nationalists, and the urban and Western-educated elite voicing claims of viewing Indian medicine as scientific. Revisiting the pristine heritage of India became the sole aim in their move toward envisioning a liberated India. To this effect, *Ayurveda* fitted into the nationalist debates of a framework of scientific rationality within a rich cultural heritage.

The establishment of a formal system of medical education in Britain, and hence of State employ, aimed to distinguish between a 'trained' and an 'untrained' doctor. The same policy, when applied to India had different implications. English or Western education was confined to the Indian middle classes, and as nationalism intensified, they produced an overt threat to British dominion. Most proposals for popularizing Western-style education owed much to the influence of Lord Macaulay who conceived of a "public service confined in its upper reaches to gentlemen of breeding and culture selected by a literary competition."[6] Further impetus to making this policy a reality was provided by Hindu College the founders of which, in trying to help promote and cultivate European sciences and literature, acted as agents of cultural transplant of secular colonial values on Indian soil. In this respect, they formed a close alliance with the Orientalist ideals of viewing Western education as a means to catalyze and reform indigenous culture and institutions; the College seen in its entirety as an "institution that acted as a key socialization agency for...[an] earlier generation of bhadralok,"[7] also exhibited "an extreme example of the working of the educational ideology"[8] in British India.

Here are some of the leading contentions of this work. Professional autonomy is an absolutely essential factor for a body of knowledge to flourish in terms of its research and experimental activities. Since these activities take place in a social and political *milieu*, the challenge to medicine by the ruling authority or the State denies this autonomy, limiting its scope of initiatives and development of scientific research. When the defense of medicine in ancient times violated the practical norms of the hierarchical society, medical practitioners came under strong condemnation by the priestly ideology, which did not accept the scientific and inquisitive mind of *Ayurvedic* physicians; for their medical knowledge was based on thousands of years of research work by medical sages. As a result, Indian medicine was seen by the earlier orthodoxy as repudiating the scriptural declarations which justified priestly laws. The only way its practitioners could tone down the intensity of such 'hostility' was by sacrificing their scientific prerogatives to political necessities which ultimately altered the nature of medical discoveries. Some of them were seen in the literary writings of medical men who "inserted appropriate qualifying remarks and disclaimers in the text to lead to rapid relaxation of the ruling against their books."[9] In line with these developments and concessions, in Europe, Copernicus dedicated his *De Revolutionibus* to Pope Paul III, while Galileo, suspected of heresy for developing a new philosophy of science that threatened the order of the universe, sought to alter the contents of the *Sunspot Letters,* at the same time resolving tensions between science and the Bible.[10] In addition, medicine is such a practical body of knowledge, as any other science, that its success depends upon the existence of a support-base or 'savior' which would advocate its freedom in practice. If professions are seen as "monopolistic bodies seeking to regulate market conditions in their favour in face of competition from outsiders,"[11] then these conditions were amply provided by the middle classes and the nobility. Once again, this limits the relevance of political patronage in encouraging the growth of a medical and scientific discipline. At least, under Muslim rule, we have no evidence of political authority demanding political and religious concessions to accept the defense of medical science, although medical compendia were, on occasions, dedicated to the reigning personages. This was also a corollary to the personal interest of the State which has led us to conclude that if there is 'scientific resonance' between the scientific community and the State, the chances of 'scientific jeopardy' are minimal. To view this as simple accretions will not do justice to medical essentials under pre-colonial India. However, judged by Kuhn's ideas of progress, each generation of *hakims* and *vaids* built up on the inherited knowledge from previous generations. While science, including medicine, progresses through continuous discoveries, argumentations of knowledge and research methods intelligible to the scientific community, its success as a practicing art was determined by the presence of a social group of consumers and patrons. And when the imperial machinery collapsed first under the Muslim rule, then the British, patrons of medicine were liquidated, thus overthrowing the support base and a willing clientele.

When the British went to India, they carried with them an assortment of clinical successes that put medicine on a sound footing through visible developments in medical practice and the overall organization of the medical profession. By the time they established their empire, these developments coupled with the new position of the literary medical tradition and practice following the Age of Renaissance, were seen as 'new' or scientific medicine. This must have been a precursor to British rejection of most theories of indigenous medical science. After all, the nature of British imperialism, its policies and impact, changed with the changing pattern in social, economic and political development in its parent country. With changes in medical concepts and practices, and the emergence of specialized disciplines which became rapid in the aftermath of the Second World War, the doctors' power and their knowledge came to rest more "on a degree of trade-off between technicality and indeterminacy, the former emphasizing the solid scientific basis of medicine, the latter stressing the interpretive mysteries of diagnosis and treatment."[12] A 'policy transplant' and cultural intrusions did not carry much favor with the Indian population. One consequence of this was the anti-colonial consciousness, intensified by the rise of the nationalist movement, the loss of monopolistic power of Western medicine, and the creation of social and political awareness amongst the intellectuals and the middle classes; the latter sought "to challenge and deny the pretended supremacy of the culture of the colonizer as well as to reassert the cultural identity of the colonized,"[13] to an extent that the real challenge for the British shifted from controlling India to framing policies that would subvert the increasing, and perhaps threatening, influence of the Western-educated elites. The introduction and imposition of Western culture and ideas, also created a 'polarized' division in the Indian masses with mixed opinions about the British rule. While some reacted with much criticism, others welcomed new opportunities of alliance with their Western counterparts. Acceptability and rejection characterized the duality in their relationship.

In studying the trajectories of Indian medicine over a period of several invasions, thus, a portrayal of the role of the intellectuals, the new middle classes, and elites as patrons of medical knowledge has been a major contention. Added to this is our belief that this study has resulted in a study of power relations between the social classes and the State in a framework of medical encounter. In view of this, if my work elicits further interest in studies on the patronage systems in a society with plural medical systems, it will fulfill the purpose for which it was intended.

Notes

Chapter 1

1. William Osler, *The Growth of Truth As Illustrated In the Discovery of the Circulation of the Blood: Selected Writings of Sir William Osier* (Oxford, 1906), 205–36.
2. Thomas S. Kuhn, *The Structure of Scientific Revolutions* (University of Chicago Press: Chicago and London, 3rd edition, 1996), 1–2.
3. Kuhn, *The Structure of Scientific Revolutions* (Chicago: Chicago University Press, 1962).
4. Richard J. Blackwell, "Approaches to the Explanation of Discovery in Science," in *Philosophy and Science as Modes of Knowing: Selected Essays,* ed., Alden L. Fisher and George B. Murray (New York: Appleton-Century-Crofts, 1969), 62–73,70.
5. Blackwell, "Approaches," 62–73.
6. Joseph Needham, *The Grand Titration: Science and Society in East and West* (London: Allen and Unwin, 1966 and 1969), 183. See also Joseph Needham, ed., *Science and Civilization in China* (Cambridge, Cambridge University Press, 1954–95). See also O.P. Jaggi, "Introduction" to *History of Science, Philosophy and Culture in Indian Civilization, General ed.,* D. P. Chattopadhyaya (Delhi: Oxford University Press), *Series,* IX, pt. I, iii–xxii.
7. Waltraud Ernst, "Plural Medicine, Tradition and Modernity-Historical and Contemporary Perspectives: Views from Below and from Above," in *Plural Medicine, Tradition and Modernity, 1800–2000,* ed., Waltraud Ernst (London: Routledge, 2002), 1–18,8.
8. Felix Marti-Ibanez, ed., *Henry Sigerist On the History of Medicine* (New York: MD Publications, Inc., 1960), 27.
9. Roy Porter and W. F. Bynum, "The Art and Science of Medicine," in *Companion Encyclopedia of the History of Medicine,* ed., Roy Porter and W.F. Bynum (London: Routledge, 1993), vol. 1,3–11, 3.
10. Porter and Bynum, "Art and Science of Medicine," 8.
11. Deborah Lupton, *Medicine as Culture: Illness, Disease and the Body in Western Societies* (Sage: London, 1994), 21. See also N. Scheper-Huges and M.M. Lock, "The Mindful Body: A Proleomenon to future work in Medical Anthropology," *Medical Anthropology Quarterly,* 1, (1987): 6–41, 8.
12. Lupton, *Medicine as Culture,* 10–11.
13. David Arnold, ed. *Imperial Medicine and Indigenous Societies* (Manchester: University Press, 1988).
14. Roger Jeffery, *The Politics of Health in India* (Berkeley: University Press, 1988).
15. Mark Harrison, *Public Health in British India: Anglo-Indian Preventive Medicine, 1859–1914* (Cambridge: University Press, 1994).

16. This was highlighted in my earlier study. Poonam Bala, *Imperialism and Medicine in Bengal: Socio-Historical Perspectives* (New Delhi: Sage, 1991).

17. See details in Kuhn, 1962.

18. Jaggi, *History of Science,* 26–7.

19. Marti-Ibanez, *History of Medicine,* xviii.

20. Marti-Ibanez, *History of Medicine,* xvii.

21. W.F. Bynum, *Science and the Practice of Medicine in the Nineteenth Century* (Cambridge: University Press, 1994).

22. Roy Porter, *The Greatest Benefit of Mankind: A Medical History of Humanity from Antiquity to the Present* (London: Harper Collins, 1997).

23. Romila Thapar, "Interpretations of Indian History: Colonial, Nationalist, and Post-colonial" (opening address given at the conference on Contemporary India in Transition, Lisbon, June 1998), 25–36, 27.

24. Arturo Castiglioni, *A History of Medicine* (New York: Knopf, 1941).

25. Debiprasad Chattopadhyaya, "Case for a Critical Analysis of the Caraka-Samhita," in *Studies in the History of Science in India,* ed., Debiprasad Chattopadhyaya (New Delhi: Editorial Enterprises, 1982), 1, 209–38, 209.

26. See details in Arnold, *Imperial Medicine.*

27. Paul C. Winther, *Anglo-European Science and the Rhetoric of Empire: Malaria, Opium, and British Rule in India, 1756–1895 (New* York: Lexington Books, 2003).

28. Benjamin Zachariah, "Uses of Scientific Argument: The Case of 'Development in India,' c!930–1950," *Economic and Political Weekly* (Sept 29, 2001): 3689–702.

29. See Deepak Kumar, ed., *Science and Empire: Essays in the Indian Context (1700–1947)* (Delhi: Anamika, 1991).

30. Mitchell Weiss, Alex Cohen, and Leon Eisenberg, "Mental Health," in *International Public Health: Diseases, Programs, and Policies,* eds., Michael H. Merson, Robert E. Black, and Anne J. Mills (Maryland: Aspen Publishers, 2001), 331–77.

31. W. Anderson, "Immunities of Empire: Race, Disease and the New Tropical Medicine, 1900–1920," *Bulletin of the History of Medicine* 70 (1996):94–118. See also Mark Harrison, "The Tender Frame of Man: Disease, Climate and Racial Difference in India and the West Indies, 1760–1860," *Bulletin of the History of Medicine* 70 (1996): 68–93.

32. Eliot Friedson, *Professionalism Reborn: Theory, Prophecy, and Policy* (Chicago: University of Chicago Press, 1994), 68–9.

33. Arthur Kleinman, *Writing at the Margin: Discourse between Anthropology and Medicine* (Berkeley: University of California Press, 1995), 22–3.

34. D. P. Chattopadhyaya, *Science and Society in Ancient India* (Calcutta: Research India Publications, 1977).

35. Claudia Liebeskind, "Arguing Science: Unani *tibb,* Hakims and Biomedicine in India, 1900–50," in *Plural Medicine, Tradition,* ed., Ernst, 58–75.

36. Charles Leslie, *Asian Medical Systems: A Comparative Study* (Berkeley: University of California, 1976).

37. Leslie. *Asian Medical Systems,* 239–41.

38. David Arnold, *Colonizing the Body: State Medicine and Epidemic Disease in 19th-Century India* (Berkeley: University of California, 1993).

39. Roger Jeffery, "Policies towards Indigenous Healers in Independent India," *Social Science and Medicine,* 16 (1982): 1835–41, 1837.

Chapter 2

1. William Jones, "Discourse on the Institution of a Society," *Asiatic Researches* xi (1788) quoted in D. Chowry Muthu, *The Antiquity of Hindu Medicine and Civilisation* (New York: Paul Hoeber, 1931), 17.
2. Gregory L. Possehl, *Indus Age: The Beginnings* (Philadelphia: University of Pennsylvania Press, 1999), 38–154. See also Jonathan Mark Kenoyer, *Ancient Cities of the Indus Valley Civilization* (Karachi: Oxford University Press, 1998).
3. Kenneth Zysk, *Religious Healing in the Vedas, Transactions of the American Philosophical Society* (Philadelphia: The American Philosophical Society, 1985), vol. 75. no. 7, 2.
4. Zysk, *Religious Healing.*
5. Herman Kulke and Dietmar Rothermund, *A History of India* (London: Routledge, 1990), 1930–33.
6. Gregory L. Possehl, ed., *Ancient Cities of the Indus* (North Carolina: Carolina Academic Press, 1979), 287–326. See also Zysk, *Religious Healing,* 4.
7. Romila Thapar, "Imagined Religious Communities? Ancient History and the Modem Search for a Hindu Identity" in *History and Beyond,* ed., Romila Thapar (New Delhi: Oxford University Press, 2000): 60–88, 82.
8. Zysk, *Religious Healing, 3*
9. Zysk, *Religious Healing,* 8.
10. Henry Sigerist, *A History of Medicine* (New York: Oxford University Press, 1961) vol. II, 161.
11. S. N. Sen, "A Survey of Source Materials," in *A Concise History of Science in India,* ed., D. M. Bose (New Delhi: Indian National Science Academy, 1971), 16.
12. *Rgveda,* 9.112.1 quoted in Zysk, *Religious Healing,* 9.
13. Muthu, *Antiquity of Hindu Medicine,* 17. See also Zysk, *Religious Healing,* 8.
14. Muthu, *Antiquity of Hindu Medicine,* 14.
15. Muthu, *Antiquity of Hindu Medicine,* 14.
16. Muthu, *Antiquity of Hindu Medicine,* 15.
17. Zysk, *Religious Healing,* 11.
18. *Mahabharata,* 66 quoted in Muthu, *Antiquity of Hindu Medicine,* 19.
19. Medical practitioners using herbs for cure of treatment, a term which later changed to *vaid,* or an *Ayurvedic* physician.
20. *Mahabharata,* chapter 84 quoted in Muthu, *Antiquity of Hindu Medicine,* 21–2.
21. D. P. Chattopadhyaya, *Science and Society in Ancient India* (Calcutta: Research India Publications, 1977).
22. J. R. Haldar, *Medical Science in Pali Literature* (Calcutta, 1977), 1.
23. Chattopadhyaya, *Science and Society in Ancient India.*
24. J. Filliozat, *The Classical Doctrine of Indian Medicine* (New Delhi: Oriental Publishers, 1964).
25. G. Jan Meulenbeld, "Reflections on the Basic Concepts of Indian Pharmacology," in *Studies on Indian Medical History,* eds., G. Jan Meulenbeld and Dominik Wujastyk (Groningen: Egbert Forsten, 1987), 1–17, 2.
26. Kenneth Zysk, "Mantra in Ayurveda: A Study of the Use of Magico-Religious Speech in Ancient India," in *Understanding Mantra,* ed., Harvey Alper (New York: SUNY Press, 1985).
27. Kuhn, 1970.

28. Kuhn, 1970.

29. Ernst Nagel, *Teleology Revisited and Other essays in the Philosophy and History of Science* (New York: Columbia University Press, 1974), 66–7.

30. Karl Popper, *Conjectures and Refutations* (New York: Basic Books, 1963), 27.

31. W. H. S. Jones, *Philosophy and Medicine in Ancient Greece* (Baltimore: The Johns Hopkins University Press, 1946).

32. Julius Jolly, *Indian Medicine,* trans. C. G. Kashikar, 2nd rev. ed. (New Delhi: Munshiram Manoharlal, 1977), 56–7.

33. Chattopadhyaya, *Science and Society.*

34. R. C. Majumdar, "Medicine," in *A History of Science,* ed., Bose, 213–68.

35. *Verse Sa.:I,* quoted by Meulenbeld in *Indian Medical History,* ed., Meulenbeld and Wujastyk, 1–15, 3 and 5.

36. For details on the theory *of Karma,* see M.G. Weiss, "Caraka Samhita on the Doctrines of Karma," *in Karma and Rebirth in the Indian Classical Tradition,* ed., W. D. O'Flaherty (Berkeley: University of California Press, 1980), 90–115.

37. *Sruti,* a Sanskrit word representing knowledge through 'what is heard.' It connotes something that was directly heard from God, by the sages, and thus based on the spiritual experience of the ancient seers through years of deep meditation.

38. *Smriti* connotes that which was written down and remembered. *Smritis* are the repository of *Dharmasastras* which laid down laws that govern Hindu society, and defined the expected conduct of a man in different stages of his life.

39. S. Radhakrishnan, *Indian Philosophy,* 1923, I, 271–76, quoted in D. P. Chattopadhyaya, *Lokayata: A Study in Ancient Indian Materialism* (New Delhi: People's Publishing House, 1959).

40. Meulenbeld in *Indian Medical History,* ed., Meulenbeld and Wujastyk, 4.

41. *Prabhava* refers to a specific action of a medicinal herb or plant.

42. Jones, *Philosophy and Medicine,* 23 and 27.

43. Almaceon is known for his pioneering work in pure medical science; his work on the anatomy remains significant even to this day.

44. Jones, *Philosophy and Medicine,* 33.

45. *Samhita* refers to a compendium.

46. Frank John Ninivaggi, *An Elementary Textbook of Ayurveda* (Madison: Psychosocial Press, 2001), 17.

47. One of the ages *ofyugas,* or periods in human history, represented by *Satya Yuga* (Golden Age), *Treta Yuga* (Silver Age), *Dvapar* (Copper Age), and *Kal Yuga* (Iron Age) or the contemporary era.

48. S. N. Dasgupta, *A History of Indian Philosophy* (Delhi: Motilal Banarsidass, 1975), vol. 1, 273. Also quoted in Antonella Comba, "Caraka Samhita, Sarirasthana I and Vaisesika Philosophy," in *Studies on History of Science,* ed., Meulenbeld and Wujastyk, 43–61.

49. E. H. Johnston, *Early Samkhya* (Delhi: Motilal Banarsidass, 1974), 10.

50. See also S. Radhakrishnan, *Indian Philosophy* (New York: MacMillan Company, 1962), 37.

51. D. S. Gaur and L. P. Gupta, "The Theory of *Pancamahabhuta* with Special Reference to *Ayurveda,*" *Indian Journal of History of Science,* no. V (1970): 51–67. See also S. K. Mishra, "Tradition of Ayurveda: Evolution and Growth," in *A Concise History,* ed., Bose, 309–15.

52. Jolly, *Indian Medicine,* 56–7.

53. K. R. Srikanta Murthy, "Salyatantra (Surgery)," in *A Concise History,* ed., Bose, 325–35.

54. Thorwald Jurgeon quoted in Murthy, "Salyatantra."

55. H. H. Sir Bhagvat Sinh Jee, *A Short History of Aryan Medical Science* (London: MacMillan & Co., 1896).

56. Debiprasad Chattopadhyaya, *Science and Society in Ancient India* (Amsterdam: B. R. Gruner, 1978).

57. Chattopadhyaya, *Science and Society,* 1977, 3.

58. Chattopadhyaya, *Science and Society,* 1977, 155.

59. H. T. Colebrooke, *Miscellaneous Essays* (London), 1837, quoted by Chattopadhyaya, 1977, 13.

60. *Susruta Samhita,* quoted by Chattopadhyaya, *Science and Society,* 1977, 97.

61. Meulenbeld in Meulenbeld and Wujastyk, 1987, 4.

62. These were born in violation of mating laws between a higher caste and *ambashthas* or *shudras.*

63. Chattopadhyaya, *Science and Society,* 1977, 36–7.

64. Chattopadhyaya, *Science and Society,* 1977, 37–8.

65. Vivian Mutton, "Healers in the Medical Market Place: Towards a Social History of Greco-Roman Medicine," in *Medicine in Society: Historical Essays,* ed., Andrew Wear (Cambridge: Cambridge University Press, 1992), 15–58, 16.

66. It is often assumed by most scholars that Greek medical knowledge diffused throughout the ancient world to become the basis for all subsequent developments and that the elements of Indian medicine were borrowed from Greek science. Filliozat, a leading French Sanskritist, argues that Indian and Greek medical traditions developed along parallel lines. Indian medicine spread to Central and South-east Asia with the spread of Buddhism.

67. B. Farrington, *Head and Hand in Ancient Greece: Four Studies in the Social Relations of nought* (London: Watts, 1947), 29.

68. Chattopadhyaya, *Science and Society,* 1977, 246.

69. Chattopadhyaya, *Science and Society,* 1977, 257.

70. Chattopadhyaya, *Science and Society,* 1977, 213.

71. *Dvijas,* or twice-born castes represented by *Brahmins. Vaishayas* and *Kshatriyas.*

72. Chattopadhyaya and Winternitz, quoted by Chattopadhyaya, *Science and Society,* 1977, 223.

73. For details, see Childe in Vijay Kumar Thakur, *Urbanisation in Ancient India* (Delhi: Abhinav Publications, 1981), 6.

74. See Richard Davis, "Introduction," in *Religions of India in Practice,* ed., Donald S. Lopez (Princeton: The University Press, 1995), 1–52.

75. Vijay Kumar Thakur, *Towns in Pre-Modern India* (New Delhi: Janaki Prakashan, 1994), 2.

76. Thakur, 1981, 196.

77. For details, sec Thakur, 1981.

78. Ninivaggi, *Textbook ofAyurveda.* 14–5. See also K.G. Zysk, *Asceticism and Healing in Ancient India: Medicine in the Buddhist Monastery* (New Delhi: Oxford University Press, 1991), 41.

79. "Academy," August 15, 1891, 138–39 in *Journal of the Pali Text Society,* ed., T. W. Rhys Davids (London: Henry Frowderc, 1893).

80. See details in Rhys Davids, *Pali Text Society,* 66.

81. *Avatar* or re-incarnation of God, according to Hindu beliefs.

82. Ninivaggi, *Textbook of Ayurveda,* 15.
83. *Ayurveda* was introduced into Tibet around 650 A.D. See also Ninivaggi, *Text book of Ayurveda.*
84. See A. F. R. Hoernle, "The Bower Manuscript," in *Studies in the History of Science in India,* ed., Debiprasad Chattopadhyaya, (Delhi: Editorial Enterprises, 1982), I, 116–140.
85. Thakore Saheb, *History of Aryan Medical Science,* 189, cited by Muthu, Antiquity of Hindu Medicine.
86. K. Chen, *Buddhism in China* (Princeton: Princeton University Press, 1984).
87. Ninavaggi, *Textbook of Ayurveda,* 20.
88. Poonam Bala, "Indigenous Medicine and the State in Ancient India," *Ancient Science of Life 5,* no. 1 (1985): 1–4.
89. Chattopadhyaya, *Science and Society,* 425.
90. L. Joshi, *Studies in the Buddhistic Culture of India* (Delhi: Motilal Banarsidass, 1964), 392.
91. Bala, "Indigenous Medicine."
92. Poonam Bala, *Imperialism and Medicine in Bengal: A Socio-Historical Perspective* (New Delhi: Sage, 1991).

Chapter 3

1. George Sarton, cited by S. M. Razaullah Ansari and Zia Fatima, "An Essay-Review on Science and Technology in Medieval India," *Studies in History of Medicine* (1984): 1–2, 67–87, 68.
2. A. Rahman, *The Cultural and Philosophical Roots of Scientific Traditions* (Delhi: National Institute of Science, Technology and Development Studies, 1983), 25. See also Ansari, 1984, 69.
3. See I. H. Qureshi, *History of the Muslim community in the Indian Subcontinent,* Ch. I, 1962, cited by Percival Spear, *A History of India* (Middlesex: Penguin Books, 1985), vol. 2, 221.
4. Spear, *History of India,* 20–21.
5. Practitioners of *Unani* medicine are also called *hakims.*
6. *Unani* medicine is also called *Unani-Tibb* by some, to indicate its Ionian origins.
7. Ninivaggi, *Textbook of Ayurveda.* 21.
8. O. P. Jaggi, *Medicine in India: Modern Period* (Delhi: Oxford University Press, 2000), 319.
9. Ninivaggi, *Textbook of Ayurveda.*
10. S. L. Bhatia, *A History of Medicine* (Delhi: Medical Council of India, 1977), 109.
11. They were Christian sectarians. Bhagavat Sinh Jee (Thakore Saheb of Golconda), *A Short History of Aryan Medical Science* (London: MacMillan and Company, 1896), 123.
12. Edwarde G. Browne, *Arabian Medicine* (Cambridge: Cambridge University Press, 1921). See also Bhatia, *History of Medicine,* 111.
13. Ninivaggi, *Textbook of Ayurveda,* 22.
14. T. Siddiqui, "Unani Medicine in India," *Indian Journal of History of Science* 16, no. 1 (May 1981): 22–25, 23.
15. R. L. Verma and N. H. Keswani, "Women in the Arabic Medicine," *Studies in the History of Medicine* (Dec.1977): 271–284, 275.
16. Jaggi, *Medicine in India,* 320.

17. M. Z. Siddiqui, "The Unani-Tibb (Greek Medicine) in India," in *A Concise History,* ed., Bose, 272.

18. N. H. Keswani, *"Medical Education in India since Ancierit Times"* (paper presented at the International Symposium, California, 1968), 59.

19. Keswani, *"MedicalEducation,"*62.

20. Keswani, *"Medical Education,"* 59.

21. Keswani, *"Medical Education,"* 1968. See also Sen et al, pp. 133–34 in Ansari, op. cit).

22. Jaggi, *Medicine in India.*

23. Jaggi, *Medicine in India,* 320. See also T.Siddiqui, "Unani Medicine in India," 18–24.

24. T. Siddiqui, "Unani Medicine in India," 1980: 22.Takas was the currency of India used in ancient and medieval times.

25. Tariq Farivaris, III, 395, cited by Bhatia, *History of Medicine,* 119.

26. Francois Bernier, *Travels in the Moghul Empire, AD 1658–1668* (Delhi: S. Chand, 1968 (original 1891), 338. See also Bernier in Zaheer Baber, *The Science of Empire: Scientific Knowledge, Civilization, and Colonial Rule in India* (Albany: State University of New York Press, 1996), 78.

27. Cited in Jaggi, *Medicine in India,* 320.

28. M. Z. Siddiqui, "The Unani-Tibb (Greek Medicine) in India," 1971: 271.

29. R. L. Verma and N. H. Keswani, "Unani Medicine in Medieval India: Its Teachers and Texts," in N. H. 'Keswani, *The Science of Medicine and Physiological Concepts in Ancient and Medieval India* (New Delhi: S. K. Manchanda, 1974), 127–42, 131.

30. Jaggi, *Medicine in India,* 321.

31. Barbara D.Metcalf, "Nationalist Muslims in British India: The Case of Hakim Ajmal Khan," *Modern Asian Studies* 19, no. 1 (1985): 1–28, 5.

32. O. P. Jaggi, *Medicine in Medieval India* (Delhi: Atma Ram, 1977), 144.

33. Verma and Keswani, "Unani Medicine," 133.

34. Hakim Abdul Fatah Gilani is known for his invention of the Indian *hookah.*

35. *Jaggi, Medicine in India,* 321.

36. Mahmud Ali and Ali Gilani, Jami-ul-Sharhain, 1848 (Arabic), cited by Verma and Keswani, "Unani Medicine," 134.

37. M. Athar Ali, "The Perception of India in Akbar and Abu'l Fazl," in *Akbar and his India,* ed., Irfan Habib (Delhi: Oxford University Press, 1997), 215–24, 215.

38. Ali," Perception of India," 222.

39. See M. A. Alavi and A.Rahman, *Shah Fat'nullah Shirazi, a 16th-century Indian Scientist* (New Delhi, 1976), cited by Iqbal Ghani Khan, "Scientific Concepts in Abul Fazl's Ain-I Akbari," in Habib, *Akbar and his India,* 121–28,128.

40. K. Chandpuri, "Fawaid Al-Insan: A Rare Manuscript of Akbar's time," *Studies in History of Medicine* I, no. 2 (1977):122–28,122.

41. Chandpuri, "Fawaid Al-Insan." See also Badauni, Muntakhab'ut Tawarikh, III. Ed. Ahmad Ali, Calcutta, 1869, p. 165, cited by Shreen Moosvi, An Estimate of Revenues of the Decca Kingdoms, 1591," in *Akbar and his India,* ed., Habib, 288–93, 289.

42. F. E. Keay, *Ancient Indian Education,* 122, cited by Edwardes and Garrett, *Mughal Rule in India* (Delhi: S. Chand and Company, 1956), 226–227.

43. Ain-i-Akbari, vol. I, p.279 trans. Blochman, cited in Edwardes and Garrett, *Mughal Rule,* 1956:227.

44. Edwardes and Garrett, *Mughal Rule,* 1956: 44.

45. Ali in *Akbar and His India,* ed., Habib, 1997:220.

46. Francoise 'Nalini' Delvoye, "The Image of Akbar as Patron of Music in Indo-Persian and Vernacular Sources," in *Akbar and His India,* ed., Habib, 188–214, 202.

47. Delvoye, "The Image of Akbar," 203.

48. R. H. Major, *A History of Medicine* (Oxford: Blackwell, 1954), 81.

49. John F. Richards, *The New Cambridge History of India: The Mughal Empire,* Cambridge: Cambridge University Press, 1993), 19.

50. Jaggi, *Medicine in India,* 321.

51. Saiyid Ahmad, ed., *Tuzuk-e-Jahangiri, Ghazipur andAligar (1863–64).* See de tails in I. Habib. *Agrarian System of Mughal India: 1556–1707* (Delhi: Oxford University Press, 1999), 115.

52. Richards, *New Cambridge History,* 104.

53. Tarapada Mukherjee and Irfan Habib, "Akbar and the Temples of Mathura and its *Environs," Proceedings of the Indian History Congress, 48th"Session.* Goa, 1987, 234–50.

54. O. P. Jaggi, *Medicine in Medieval India,* 181.

55. Richards, *The New Cambridge History,* 152.

56. Richards, *The New Cambridge History,* 161.

57. Verma and Keswani, "Unani Medicine, "138.

58. Richards, *The New Cambridge History,* 173.

59. Verma and Keswani, *"Unani Medicine,"* 139.

60. I. A. Khan, "The Middle Classes in the Mughal Empire," *Social Scientist 5,* no. 1, (1977): 28–49,28.

61. A characteristic feature of economy in medieval India was the existence of the feudal mode of production. This meant that the subordinate classes were linked to the State and local government through various intermediaries and feudal lords.

62. Moreland, cited by Khan, "The Middle Classes," 37.

63. Plural of *waqf.*

64. Habib, *Agrarian System,* 12.

65. Habib, *Agrarian System,* 358.

66. See the preamble of Aurangzeb's *farman of 1690,* Allahabad II, 53 & 55 cited by Habib, *Agrarian System, 352* fn 48).

67. Habib, *Agrarian System,* 352–353.

68. S. H. Hodivala, *Studies in Parsi History* (Bombay, 1920), 149–88, 178.

69. Habib, *Agrarian System, (farman* or royal decree).

70. Practitioners *of Ayurveda,* also called *vaids.*

71. Holders of special ranks or *mansab* bestowed by the emperor in recognition of special services.

72. Holders or assignees *of jagir* or land assigned by the emperor.

73. Khan, "The Middle Classes."

74. Khan, "The Middle Classes," 40.

75. See Habib, *Agrarian System,* 355.

76. Richards, *The New Cambridge History,* 91–3.

77. See Badauni cited by Habib, *Agrarian System,* 358.

78. Khan, "The Middle Classes," 31.

79. Khan, "The Middle Classes,"31.

80. K. N. Raj, "Politics and Economics of Intermediate Regimes," *Economic and Political Weekly* viii, no.27 (7 July 1973): 1191.

81. Khan, "The Middle Classes," 32.

82. Richards, *The New Cambridge History,* 149–50.

83. See Balkrishan Brahman's letter to a relation contained in the collection of Maktubat MS, add. 16859. Details in Khan, "The Middle Classes."

84. See Moreland, *India at the Death of Akbar* (1972): 79 in Khan "The Middle Classes," 37.

85. Muslim judge.

86. Niccolao Manucci, *Storio Do Mogor or Mughal India, 1653–1708,* trans. William Irvine, II (London, 1907), 176,179, and 214–227. Also see Khan, "The Middle Classes," 38.

87. Habib, *Agrarian System.*

88. Khan, "The Middle Classes," 38.

89. Khan, "The Middle Classes," 39.

90. Landholders.

91. Muzafiar Alam, *The Crisis of Empire in North India* (Delhi: Oxford University Press, 1986), 1.

92. *Jagir* was an area whose revenue was assigned by the emperor.

93. Femard Braudel, *Civilization and Capitalism, 15th–18th-Century: The Perspective of the World* (London: William Collins, 1984), vol.3, 513. See also Baber, *Science of Empire.*

94. Manrique, cited by Habib, *Agrarian System,* 370.

95. Local prince.

96. For details, see Khan, "The Middle Classes," 1977:40.

97. Irfan Habib, "Colonisation of the Indian Economy," *Social Scientist* 3 (1975): 22–53, 42.

98. *Muquaddam* is an Arabic word which means 'one who is placed first.' In medieval times, however, the term came to be used for the village headman in North India (equivalent to Patel in South India or Dakhin).

99. *Mahal* is the unit for revenue purposes or *parganas,* which marks the territory delimited by Mughal administration for revenue and administrative purposes.

100. Holders *of miras,* or hereditary land allotment.

101. Habib, "Colonisation of the Indian Economy," 26.

102. Habib, "Colonisation of the Indian Economy."

103. A. W. Zahuri. "Development of Greco-Arab Literature in India," *Studies in History of Medicine* iii, no.2 (1979):125– 45,125.

104. A. Rahman. "Science and Technology in Medieval India: Introduction to a Bibliography of Source Material in Sanskrit, Arabic and Persian," *Cressida Transactions* 1, no. 1 (1981):187–98, 195.

105. T. Siddiqui, "Unani Medicine in India during the Delhi Sultanate," *Studies in History of Medicine* II, no.3 (1978): 183–89,184.

106. Kuhn, *Structure of Scientific Revolutions,* 1970. Paradigm is a specific theory, law etc., based on the achievements of a scientific community, and provides a framework for solving scientific puzzles. This framework does not change as long as solutions to puzzles continue to be resolved. If it does not, it is replaced in whole or in part by a new one which Kuhn calls a 'revolution' in science.

107. P. Kutumbiah, *Ancient Indian Medicine* (Madras: V. Abdullah, 1962), xliv.

108. Keswani in Verma and Keswani, "Unani Medicine," 61.

109. A. H. Israili, "Education of Unani Medicine during Mughal Period," *Studies in History of Medicine* IV, no.3 (1980): 177–82, 180.

110. A. Jalil, "The Evolution of Development of Greco-Arab Medical Education," *Studies in History of Medicine* ii, no.3 (1978): 190–97, 195.

111. Jalil, "Greco-Arab Medical Education," 196.

112. M. Z. Siddiqui, "The Unani-Tibb (Greek Medicine) in Indja," 272.

113. Satish Chandra, *Parties and Politics at the Mughal Court. 1707–1740* (Delhi, Oxford University Press, 2002), 13.

114. Chandra, *Parties and Politics.*

Chapter 4

1. Court of Directors, *Public Disputations,* 1814, 5. See also David Kopf, *British Orientalism and Bengal Renaissance: The Dynamics of Indian Modernization, 1773–1835* (Berkeley: University of California Press, 1969), 152–53.

2. J. N. Sarkar, ed., *Later Mughals,* 311, cited by S. M. Edwards and H.L.O. Garrett. *Mughal Rule in India.*

3. Michael Edwardes, *British India, 1773–1947: A Survey of the Nature and Effects of Alien Rule* (New York: Taplinger Publishing Company, 1968), 6.

4. One who teaches the religious teachings of Islam.

5. A. L. Basham, "The Practice of Medicine in Ancient and Medieval India," in *Asian Medical Systems: A Comparative Study,* ed., Charles Leslie (Berkeley: University of California Press, 1976), 18–43, 40.

6. Edwardes, *British India,* 11.

7. Charles Leslie, "The Ambiguities of Medical Revivalism in Modern India," in *Asian Medical Systems,* ed., Leslie, 356–67, 358.

8. Jaggi, *Medicine in Medieval India,* and Brahmananda Gupta, "Indigenous Medicine in Nineteenth-and Twentieth-Century Bengal," in *Asian Medical Systems,* ed., Leslie, 368–78.

9. Brahmananda Gupta, "Indigenous Medicine."

10. Brahmananda Gupta, "Indigenous Medicine."

11. D. G. Crawford. *History of the Indian Medical Service: 1600–1913,* vols. 1 & 2 (London: W. Thackcr, 1914).

12. Keswani, *"Medical Education,"* 65.

13. Leslie quoted by Jeffery, *Politics of Health,* 51.

14. Crawford, *History.*

15. Edwardes, *British India,* 36.

16. 'Schools' in British India referred to short courses aimed more closely at employment prospects in the subordinate medical services, as compared to 'Colleges' which prepared students for entry into the Indian Medical Services. This distinction only be came apparent after 1860 (In a personal communication with Roger Jeffery in 1982).

17. Anonymous, "Hindu Medicine and Medical Education," *Calcutta Review* 38, no. LXXXIII (1865): 106–125, 115.

18. *Medical Proceedings,* no.232 (1835), NAI.

19. Anonymous, "Hindu Medicine," 1865.

20. See details in Kopf, *British Orientalism,* fn. 11, 238.

21. Kopf, *British Orientalism,* 239.

22. "Mill's History," *Calcutta Journal* (June 20, 1819): 10–20. See also fn. in Kopf, *British Orientalism,* 240).

23. Kopf, *British Orientalism,* 202, & 270–71.

24. Keswani, *"Medical Education in India,"* 65.

25. O. P. Jaggi, "Indigenous System of Medicine during British Supremacy in India," *Studies in History of Medicine* 1, no.4 (Dec.1977): 320–41, 327.

26. K. N. Udupa, "The Health System in India," in *Health by The People,* ed., K.W. Newell (Geneva: WHO, 1975).
27. Brahmananda Gupta," Indigenous Medicine," 370.
28. Indian Medical Gazette, cited by Jaggi, *Medicine in Medieval India.*
29. Roger Jeffery, "Recognizing India's Doctors: The Institutionalization of Medical Dependency (1918–39)," *Modern Asian Studies* 13, no.2 (1979): 301–26, 320.
30. Brahmananda Gupta, "Indigenous Medicine."
31. Anil Seal, *The Emergence of Indian Nationalism* (Cambridge: Cambridge University Press, 1968), 120.
32. Brahmananda Gupta, "Indigenous Medicine."
33. Leslie quoted by Eliot Friedson and J. Lorber, *Medical Men and Their Work; A Sociological Reader,* eds., (Chicago: Aldine, 1972), 48.
34. Leslie in *Medical Men.*
35. *Bombay Record Office,* General Department, 1838, vol.21A/448A.
36. *Jeffery, Politics of Health, 55.*
37. T.J. Johnson, *Professions and Power* (London: Macmillan, 1972).
38. Crawford, *History of the Indian Medical Service.*
39. Brahmananda Gupta, "Indigenous Medicine," 371.
40. Brahmananda Gupta, "Indigenous Medicine."
41. Delhi Records 6, *Home Department Proceedings,* July 1919, Medical Branch, NAI.
42. Delhi Records 6, July 1919.
43. Brahmananda Gupta, "Indigenous Medicine."
44. *EHL,* 1919, July 26–51A, NAI.
45. O. P. Jaggi, "Indigenous Medicine during British Supremacy in India," *Studies in History of Medicine* I, no. 4 (1977): 320–47, 320.
46. Leslie, "Introduction" in Asian Medical Systems, ed., Leslie, 1–12, 7.
47. *EHL,* Sept, 1926, Health Branch, NAI.
48. Delhi Records 6, *Home Department Proceedings,* Aug. 1912, Medical Branch, NAI.
49. Katharine Park, "Medicine and Society in Medieval Europe: 500–1500," in *Medicine in Society,* ed., Andrew Wear (Cambridge: Cambridge University Press, 1992), 59–90, 75.
50. A. Wolf, *A History of Science. Technology and Philosophy in Sixteenth and Seventeenth Centuries* (Gloucester: Peter Smith, 1968), vol. II, 431.
51. Dipankar Gupta, "Knowledge and The State: A Critique of Practical Science," *Journal of Higher Education* 7, no.3 (1982):189–99.
52. L.S. King, *The Medical World of the Eighteenth Century* (New York: Robert Krieger, 1958), 264.
53. R. Richardson, *Death. Dissection and the Destitute* (London: Penguin, 1988), 32–4. See also Deborah Lupton, *Medicine as Culture: Illness, Disease and the Body in Western Societies,* London: Sage, 1994), 44–5.
54. D. Armstrong, "Silence and Truth in Death and Dying," *Social Science and Medicine,* 24, no.8, (1987): 651–57.
55. Lupton, *Medicine as Culture,* 45.
56. Richardson, *Death, Dissection and the Destitute,* 72.
57. Thomas Wise, *Commentary on the Hindu System of Medicine* (London: Trubner, 1860). See also D. Chowry Muthu, *The Antiquity of Hindu Medicine and Civilisation* (New York: Paul Hoeber, 1931), 29.

58. See also Lindsay Granshaw, "The Rise of the Modem Hospital in Britain," in *Medicine in Society, ed.*, Wear, 197–218, 206.

59. Chaasar Moir cited by Douglas Guthrie, *A History of Medicine* (New York: Thomas Nelson, 1958), 301.

60. Guthrie, *History of Medicine*, 245.

61. See E.Fisher-Homberger, "Eighteenth-Century Nosology and its Survivors," *Medical History* 14 (1970): 397–403. See also Guenther B. Risse, "Medicine in the Age of Enlightenment," in *Medicine in Society*, ed., Wear, 149–95, 167.

62. E. Goldschmid, "Nosoligia Naturalis," in E. Ashworth Underwood, ed., (London: Oxford University Press, 1953), vol. II, 104.

63. J. Filliozat, *The Classical Doctrine of Indian Medicine* (New Delhi: Oriental Publishers, 1964), 107.

64. Parke, Davis and Company, *Great Moments in Medicine-A History of Medicine in Pictures,* Stories by George A. Bender, paintings by Robert A. Thom (Detroit: Northwood Institute Press, 1966), 170–72.

65. Parke, Davis and Company, *Great Moments*, 11.

66. In 1812, a proposal was made for medical training at the Calcutta Presidency General Hospital and the General Dispensary (in a personal communication with Roger Jeffery, 1982).

67. Jeffery (in a personal communication, 1982).

68. Anonymous, "Hindu Medicine," 121.

69. David Kopf, *British Orientalism and the Bengal Renaissance: The Dynamics of Modernization, 1773–1835* (Berkeley: University of California Press, Berkeley, 1969), 241.

70. See Mill in Kopf, *British Orientalism*, 240–41. The Act excluded Indians from all higher posts.

71. H. R. Mehta, *A History of the Growth and Development of Western Education in Punjab: 1846–1886* (Punjab Government Records), 13–4.

72. See K. N. Pannikar, *Culture, Ideology, Hegemony: Intellectuals and Social Consciousness in Colonial India* (London: Anthem Press, 1995).

73. R.W. Frazer, *British India* (New Delhi: Ashish Publishers, 1974), 215.

74. Kopf, *British Orientalism*, 140.

75. Bala, *Imperialism and Medicine in Bengal.* See also Harry Cleaver, "Political Economy of Malaria De-Control," *Economic and Political Weekly* II, no. 36 (1976): 1463–73.

76. See Z. A. Nizami. *Hakim Ajmal Khan* (New Delhi, 1988), 33.

77. Bronislaw Malinowski, *A Scientific Theory of Culture and Other Essays* (New York: Oxford University Press, 1960), 43.

78. Malinowski, *Scientific Theory*, 54.

79. Wellesley went to India in 1798 as the Governor-General of Bengal. See also Kopf, *British Orientalism*, 6.

80. Kopf, *British Orientalism*, 8.

81. *Centenary Volume*, 301,303. See also Kopf, *British Orientalism*, fn. 180.

82. Kopf, *British Orientalism*, 15.

83. For details, see *The Asiatic Society (1784–1984), Bicentenary Report* (Calcutta, 1985).

84. Kopf, *British Orientalism*, 180.

85. *Sanskrit College*, General Records and Correspondence, 1827–55.

86. Kopf, *British Orientalism*, 5.

87. Kopf, *British Orientalism,* 257.

88. Traditional schools of Sanskrit learning. See detailsjn K.N.Dhar, "Old Calcutta: Its Schoolmasters," *Calcutta Review,* no. CXXXIV (July 1913): 346.

89. Kopf, *British Orientalism,* 264.

90. B. B. Patel, *Parsi,* Bombay: Prakash, vols. I–IV. Also, Hormazdyar Dastur Kayoji Mirza, *Outlines of Parsi History* (Bombay: Dastur Kayoji Mirza, 1974), 254.

91. An early record of the translation of a Sanskrit book on Indian medicine for use by Parsi priests is that of 1486.

92. Patel cited by Mirza, *Outlines of Parsi History,* 255.

93. Ashok V. Desai, "The Origins of Parsi Enterprise," in Rajat Kanta Ray. *Entrepreneurship and Industry in India: 1800–1947* (Delhi: Oxford University Press, 1992), 99–108, 106.

94. William Milburn, *Oriental Commerce.* 1813, vol.1, 124. See also Edwardes, *British India,* 90.

95. Mirza, *Outlines of Parsi History,* 1974, 256.

96. Rustomjee Naserwanjee Khory and Nanabhai Navroji Katrak, *The Bombay Materia Medica and Their Therapeutics* (Bombay: Times of India Press, 1903) Courtesy of Wellcome Institute for History of Medicine Library, London).

97. J. H. Broomfteld, *Elite Conflict in a Plural Society: Twentieth-Century Bengal* (Bombay: Oxford University Press, 1968), 12–3.

98. Bala, *Imperialism and Medicine in Bengal,* 111.

99. Broomfield, *Elite Conflict,* 1968.

100. Poonam Bala, "Ayurveda and the British Raj: Factors Influencing State Policy in British India," *Studies in History of Medicine* 8 (1984): 13–9.

101. Cleaver, "Political Economy."

102. C. R. Venkataraman, "A History of Medicine in India (1664–1945)," *Indian Journal of History of Medicine* 19, no. 1, (1974): 5–14, 5.

103. Bala, *Imperialism and Medicine in Bengal.*

104. *Proceedings of the Government of India,* Home Department, September-October, 1837.

105. Poonam Bala, "State Policy Towards Indigenous Drugs in British Bengal," *Journal of the European Ayurvedic Society* I (1990):167–76. See also Poonam Bala, "Indian and Western Medicine: Rival Traditions in British India," in *Colonialism and Psychiatry,* eds., Dinesh Bhugra and Roland Littlewood (Delhi: Oxford University Press, 2001), 232–43.

106. David Arnold, *Colonizing the Body: State, Medicine and Epidemic Disease in Nineteenth-Century India* (Berkeley: University of California Press, 1993).

107. Percival Spear, *A History of India* (Middlesex: Penguin Books, 1978).

108. Bala, "Indian and Western Medicine."

109. Bipan Chandra, ATripathi and Barun De, *Freedom Struggle* (Delhi: National Book Trust, 1972), 39.

110. Spear, *History of India,* 128.

111. Ian Copland, *India: 1885–1947: The Unmaking of an Empire, Seminar Studies in History* (Longman: Edinburgh, 2001), 34.

112. Copland, *India,* 35.

113. Edwardes, *British India,* 139.

114. *Home Department, Public A Proceedings,* no. 177 (June 1906). See also *Home Department, Public A Proceedings,* nos. 50–60 (October 1907). See also Tara Chand, *History of Freedom Movement in India,* (Delhi: Ministry of Education, 1913), vol. 3.

115. B. T. McCully, *English Education and the Origins of Indian Nationalism* (Gloucester: Peter Smith, 1966), 254.

116. McCully, *English Education,* 246.

117. Daniel Thorner, *The Shaping of Modern India* (Delhi: R.N. Sachdev, 1980), 30.

118. McCully, *English Education,* 394.

119. Francis Robinson, *Separatism among Indian Muslims: The Politics of the United Provinces Muslims, 1860–1923* (Cambridge: Cambridge University Press, 1974), 377. See also Barbara D.Metcalf, "Nationalist Muslims in British India: The Case of Hakim Ajmal Khan," *Modern Asian Studies* 19, no. 1 (1985): 1–28.

120. G. Leitner, *History of Indigenous Education in the Panjab since Annexation and in 1882* (Calcutta: Superintendent of Government Printing, 1882), 152–53. See also Jeffery, *Politics of Health,* 46–7.

121. McCully, *English Education.*

122. McCully, *English Education,* 271.

123. McCully, *English Education.*

124. Charles Leslie, "The Ambiguities of Medical Revivalism in India," in *Asian Medical Systems,* ed., Leslie, 360–61.

125. McCully, *English Education.*

126. Paul Brass," The Politics of Ayurvedic Education: A Case Study of Revivalism and Modernization in India," in *Education and Politics in India,* eds., S.H. Rudolph and LI. Rudolph (Oxford: Oxford University Press, 1972), 342–71, 344.

127. Kuhn, *The Structure of Scientific Revolutions,* 1972.

128. B.N. Pandey, *The Break-up of British India* (London: Macmillan, 1969), 32.

129. *Dawakhana* included both pharmacy and clinic. For details, see Subhuti Dharmananda, "The Ayurvedic Medicine Industry in India," *START Manuscripts* (Oregon: Institute for Traditional medicine, September 2003).

130. *Report of the All India Ayurvedic Conference, Seventh Session,* Madras, 1915.

131. *Official Correspondence,* Officiating Deputy Secretary, Government of India, to Chief Commissioner Delhi, Home, B File no.70,1920, NAI.

132. B. J. Steinthal, "The Ayurvedic Revivalist Movement in Early Twentieth-Century British India" (B.A. thesis, Harvard University, 1984).

133. Delhi Records 6, *Home Department Proceedings,* Medical Branch, July 1919, 26–51, NAI.

134. *Home/Medical Proceedings,* July 1916, A, 38–90, NAI.

135. *Home/Medical Proceedings,* July 1919, A, 2651, Proceedings 41, p.127–28, NAI.

136. Daniel Thorner, *The Shaping of Modern India* (New Delhi: R. N. Sachdev, 1980), 38.

137. *A Note on Chopra Committee's Report on Indigenous Medicine* by Dr. K.C.K.E. Raj, Director General of Health Services, 1949, 1, in *Report of Government of India Committee on Indigenous Systems of Medicine* (Chopra Committee), File 1105/1949, Medical (B) Department, Uttar Pradesh State Archives (UPSA). See also Claudia Liebeskind, "Arguing Science: Unani-tibb, hakims and biomedicine in India, 1900–50," in Ernst, *Plural Medicine,* 58–75.

138. Girindranath Mukhopadhyaya, *History of Indian Medicine* (Calcutta: University of Calcutta, 1926), vol. II.

139. Liebeskind, "Arguing Science,"63.

140. Liebeskind, "Arguing Science."

141. In 1933, Chaudhuri Rahmat Ali coined the name 'Pakistan' (land of the 'pure') for the sovereign Muslim areas he suggested should be created inside India. The word

was derived from the initial letters of the Punjab, Afghania, Kashmir and Sind with the suffix of 'tan' to represent Baluchistan. Written in Urdu language, the word is written without an 'i'. See Edwardes, British India, 294–95).

142. Brass, "The Politics of Ayurvedic Education," 359.

143. Brass, "The Politics of Ayurvedic Education," 357–8.

144. Brass, "The Politics of Ayurvedic Education."

145. *Report of the Health Survey and Planning Committee* (Delhi, 1962), vol. 1:454.

146. They were simply elaborations in urban settings of a Tol-with-a-printing press.

147. See Leslie in *Medical Men,* eds., Friedson and Lorber, 51.

148. Charles Leslie, "Modern India's Ancient Medicine," *Transaction* (June 1969): 46–55,54.

149. G. J. Hausman, "Siddhars, Alchemy and the Abyss of Tradition: 'Traditional,' Tamil Medical Knowledge in 'Modern' Practice" (Ph.D. diss., University of Michigan, 1996), 203–52.

150. Resolution no. 1 1, Adopted by the Central Provincial Health Ministers. Conference, New Delhi. See O.P.Jaggi, "Indian Systems of Medicine during British Supremacy in India," Studies in History of Medicine 1, no. 4 (June 1977): 320–47, 342.

151. *Report of the Health Survey and Development Committee* (Delhi, 1946), vol. IV, 73.

152. *Report,* 1946, vol. II, 455.

153. *Report,* 1946, vol. II, 453.

154. Brass, "The Politics of Ayurvedic Education," 252.

Conclusions

1. Chandra, Parties and Politics, 19.
2. Khan, 1977,42.
3. Blackwell, "Approaches," in Philosophy and Science, ed., Fisher and Murray, 62–73: 70.
4. Gyan Prakash, *Another Reason: Science and the Imagination of Modern India,* (Princeton: Princeton University Press, 1999), 35.
5. Liebeskind, "Arguing Science," 70.
6. See J. Donald Kingsley, *Representative Bureaucracy: An Interpretation of the British Civil Service* (Ohio: Yellow Springs, 1944), 68–71.
7. John McGuire, *The Making of a Colonial Mind: A Quantitative Study of the Bhadralok in Clacutta. 1857–1885* (Canberra: Australian National University, 1983), 47.
8. Tithi Bhattacharya, *The Sentinels of Culture: Class, Education and the Colonial Intellectual in Bengal, 1848–85* (Delhi: Oxford University Press, 2005), 175.
9. Dava Sobel, *Galileo's Daughter* (New York: Walker and Company, 1999).
10. Sobel, *Galileo's Daughter,* 159–60. See also *Letters to Father (Suor Maria Celeste) to Galileo (1623–1633),* trans, and annotated by Dava Sobel, New York: Walker and Co., 2001). The latter consists of about 124 letters Galileo's daughter wrote between 1623 and 1633, depicting an almost complete life of Galileo.
11. Mike Saks, "Removing the Blinkers? A Critique of Recent Contributions to the Sociology of Professions," Sociological Review, 1983, 31 (1): 1–21. See also David Kelleher and Gareth Williams (eds.), *Challenging Medicine* (Routledge: London and New York, 1994), xi–xxix, xii.

12. H.Jamous and B.Peloille, "Changes in the French University-Hospital System," in J.A. Jackson, ed. *Professions and Professionalization* (Cambridge: Cambridge University Press, 1970). See also David Kelleher, Jonathan Gabe and Gareth Williams, "Understanding Medical Dominance in the Modern World," in *Challenging Medicine*, xi–xxix.

13. Pannikar, *Culture, Ideology. Hegemony,* 80.

Bibliography

Alam, M. *The Crisis of Empire in North India.* Delhi: Oxford University Press, 1986.

Alavi, M. A. and A. Rahman, *Shah Fat'hullah Shirazi, a 16th-century Indian Scientist.* New Delhi, 1976.

Ali, M. A. "The Perception of India in Akbar and Abu'l Fazl." Pp.215–24 in *Akbar and his India,* edited by Irfan Habib. Delhi: Oxford University Press, 1997.

Alper, H. ed. *Understanding Mantra.* New York: SUNY Press, 1985.

Anderson, W. "Immunities of Empire: Race, Disease and the New Tropical Medicine, 1900–1920." *Bulletin of the History of Medicine* 70 (1996): 94–118.

Anonymous. "Hindu Medicine and Medical Education." *Calcutta Review* 38, no. LXXXIH (1865): 106–25.

Ansari, S. M. R. and Z. Fatim'a. "An Essay-Review on Science and Technology in Medieval India." *Studies in History of Medicine* 1–2 (1984): 67–87.

Armstrong, D. "Silence and Truth in Death and Dying," *Social Science and Medicine* 24, no. 8 (1987): 651–657.

Arnold, D. *Colonizing the Body: State, Medicine and Epidemic Disease in Nineteenth-Century India.* Berkeley: University of California Press, 1993.

——.*Imperial Medicine and Indigenous Societies.* Manchester: University Press, 1988.

Baber, Z. *The Science of Empire: Scientific Knowledge, Civilization, and Colonial Rule in India.* Albany: State University of New York Press, 1996.

Bala, P. "Ayurveda and the British Raj: Factors Influencing State Policy in British India." *Studies in History of Medicine* 8 (1984): 13–9.

——."Indian and Western Medicine: Rival Traditions in British India."Pp.232–43 in *Colonialism and Psychiatry,* edited by Dinesh Bhugra and Roland Littlewood. Delhi: Oxford University Press, 2001.

——."State Policy Towards Indigenous Drugs in British Bengal." *Journal of the European Ayurvedic Society* I (1990): 167–76.

——.*Imperialism and Medicine in Bengal: Socio-Historical Perspectives.* New Delhi: Sage, 1991.

——."Indigenous Medicine and the State in Ancient *India." Ancient Science of Life* 5, no. 1 (1985): 1–4.

Basham, A. L. "The Practice of Medicine in Ancient and Medieval India." Pp. 18–43 in *Asian Medical Systems: A Comparative Study,* edited by Charles Leslie. Berkeley: University of California Press, 1976.

Bernier, F. *Travels in the Moghul Empire, AD 1658–1668.* Delhi: S. Chand, 1968 (original 1891).

Bhattacharya, T. *The Sentinels of Culture: Class, Education and the Colonial Intellectual in Bengal, 1848–85.* Delhi: Oxford University Press, 2005.

Bhatia, S.L. *A History of Medicine.* Delhi: Medical Council of India, 1977.

Blackwell, R. J. "Approaches to the Explanation of Discovery in Science," Pp.62–73 in *Philosophy and Science as Modes of Knowing: Selected Essays,* edited by A. L. Fisher and G. B. Murray. New York: Appleton-Century Crofts, 1969.

Bombay Record Office, General Department, 1838, vol. 21A/448A.

Bose, D. M. ed. *A Concise History of Science in India.* New Delhi: Indian National Science Academy, 1971.

Brass, P. "The Politics of Ayurvedic Education: A Case Study of Revivalism and Modernization in India." Pp. 342–71 in *Education and Politics in India,* edited by S. H. Rudolph and L. I. Rudolph. Oxford: Oxford University Press, 1972.

Braudel, F. *Civilization and Capitalism,* 15th–18th *Century: The Perspective of the World.* vol 3, London: William Collins, 1984.

Broomfield, J.H. *Elite Conflict in a Plural Society: Twentieth-Century Bengal.* Bombay: Oxford University Press, 1968.

Browne, E. G. *Arabian Medicine.* Cambridge: Cambridge University Press, 1921.

Bynum, W. F. *Science and the Practice of Medicine in the Nineteenth Century.* Cambridge: University Press, 1994.

Castiglioni. A. *A History of Medicine.* New York: Knopf, 1941.

Centenary Volume, 301,303. See also Kopf, *British Orientalism,* fn, 180.

Chand, T. *History of Freedom Movement in India,* vol.3. Delhi: Ministry of Education, 1913.

Chandpuri, K. "Fawaid Al-Insan: A Rare Manuscript of Akbar's time." *Studies in History of Medicine* I, no. 2 (1977): 122–28.

Chandra, B., A. Tripathi and B. De. *Freedom Struggle.* Delhi: National Book Trust, 1972.

Chandra, S. *Parties and Politics at the Mughal Court. 1707–1740.* Delhi, Oxford University Press, 2002.

Charles L. *Asian Medical Systems: A Comparative Study.* Berkeley: University of California, 1976.

Chattopadhyaya, D.P. *Lokayata: A Study in Ancient Indian Materialism.* New Delhi: People's Publishing House, 1959.

——.*Science and Society in Ancient India.* Calcutta: Research India Publications, 1977.

——.*Science and Society in Ancient India.* Amsterdam: B.R. Gruner, 1978.

Chattopadhyaya, D. "Case for a Critical Analysis of the Caraka-Samhita," Pp. 209–38 in *Studies in the History of Science in India,* edited by Debiprasad Chattopadhyaya. Delhi: Editorial Enterprises, 1982, 1.

Chen, K. *Buddhism in China.* Princeton: Princeton University Press, 1984.

Cleaver, H. "Political Economy of Malaria De-Control." *Economic and Political Weekly* II, no.36 (1976): 1463–73.

Colebrooke, H. T. *Miscellaneous Essays.* London, 1837.

Copland, I. *India: 1885–1947: The Unmaking of an Empire: Seminar Studies in History.* Longman: Edinburgh, 2001.

Crawford, D.G. *History of the Indian Medical Service: 1600–1913,* vols. 1 & 2. London: W. Thacker, 1914.

Dasgupta, S. N. *A History of Indian Philosophy,* vol. I. Delhi: Motilal Banarsidass, 1975.

Davids, T.W. R. *Journal of the Pali Text Society.* London: Henry Frowdere, 1893.

Davis, R. "Introduction," Pp. 1–52 in *Religions of India in Practice,* edited by D.S. Lopez. Princeton: The University Press, 1995.

Delhi Records 6, *Home Department Proceedings,* Medical Branch, July 1919, 26–51, NAI.

Delhi Records 6, *Home Department Proceedings.* Aug. 1912, Medical Branch, NAI.

Delhi Records 6, *Home Department Proceedings.* July 1919, Medical Branch, NAI.

Delvoye, F.'Nalini.' "The Image of Akbar as a Patron of Music in Indo-Persian and Vernacular Sources." Pp. 188–214 in *Akbar and His India,* edited by Irfan Habib. Delhi: Oxford University Press, 1997.

Desai, A.V. "The Origins of Parsi Enterprise." Pp. 99–108 in *Entrepreneurship and Industry in India: 1800–1947,* edited by Rajat Kanta Ray. Delhi: Oxford University Press, 1992.

Dhar, K. N. "Old Calcutta: Its Schoolmasters." *Calcutta Review,* no. CXXXIV (July 1913): 346.

Dharmananda, S. "The Ayurvedic Medicine Industry in India." START Manuscripts, (Institute for Traditional Medicine, September 2003).

Education, Health and Lands, 1919, July 26–51A, NAI.

Education, Health and Lands. Sept., 1926, Health Branch, NAI.

Edwardes, M. *British India, 1773–1947: A Survey of the Nature and Effects of Alien Rule.* New York: Taplinger Publishing Company, 1968.

Ernst, W. "Plural Medicine, Tradition and Modernity-Historical and Contemporary Perspectives: Views from Below and from Above." Pp. 1–18, in *Plural Medicine, Tradition and Modernity, 1800–2000,* edited by Waltraud Ernst London: Routledge, 2002.

——.ed., Plural Medicine, Tradition and Modernity, 1800–2000. London: Routledge, 2002.

Farrington, B. *Head and Hand in Ancient Greece* (London), 1947.

Filliozat, J. *The Classical Doctrine of Indian Medicine.* New Delhi: Oriental Publishers, 1964.

Fisher, A. L. and G. B. Murray, eds. *Philosophy and Science as Modes of Knowing: Selected Essays.* New York: Appleton-Century Crofts, 1969.

Fisher-Homberger, E. "Eighteenth-Century Nosology and its Survivors." *Medical History* 14 (1970): 397–403.

Frazer, R.W. *British India.* New Delhi: Ashish Publishers, 1974.

Friedson, E. and J. Lorber, eds. *Medical Men and Their Work: A Sociological Reader.* Chicago: Aldine, 1972.

Friedson, E. *Professionalism Reborn: Theory, Prophecy, and Policy.* Chicago: University of Chicago Press, 1994.

Gaur, D. S. and L. P. Gupta. "The Theory of *Pancamahabhuta* with Special Reference to Ayurveda." *Indian Journal of History of Science,* no. v (1970): 51–67.

Granshaw, L. "The Rise of the Modem Hospital in Britain." Pp. 197–218 in *Medicine in Society,* edited by Andrew Wear. Cambridge: Cambridge University Press, 1992.

Gupta, B. "Indigenous Medicine in Nineteenth-and Twentieth-Century Bengal." Pp. 368–78 in *Asian Medical Systems: A Comparative Study,* edited by Charles Leslie. Berkeley: University of California Press, 1976.

Gupta, D. "Knowledge and the State: A Critique of Practical Science." *Journal of Higher Education* 7, no. 3 (1982): 189–99.

Guthrie, D. *A History of Medicine:* New York: Thomas Nelson, 1958.

Habib, I. "Colonisation of the Indian Economy." *Social Scientist* 3 (1975): 22–53.

Haldar, J.R. *Medical Science in Pali Literature.* Calcutta, 1977.

Harrison, M. *Public Health in British India: Anglo-Indian preventive Medicine, 1859–1914.* Cambridge: University Press, 1994.

——."The Tender Frame of Man: Disease, Climate and Racial Difference in India and the West Indies, 1760–1860," *Bulletin of the History of Medicine* 70 (1996): 68-93.

Hausman, G. J. "Siddhars, Alchemy and the Abyss of Tradition: 'Traditional,' Tamil Medical Knowledge in 'Modern' Practice" (Ph.D. dissertation, University of Michigan, 1996): 203–52.

Hodivala, S. H. *Studies in Parsi History.* Bombay, 1920.

Hoernle, A. F. R. "The Bower Manuscript." Pp. 116–140 in *Studies in the History of Science in India,* vol. 1, edited by Debiprasad Chattopadhyaya, Delhi: Editorial Enterprises, 1982.

Home Department, Public A Proceedings, no. 177 (June 1906).

Home Department, Public A Proceedings, nos. 50–60 (October 1907).

Home/Medical Proceedings, July 1916, A, 38–90, NAI.

Home/Medical Proceedings. July 1919, A, 2651, Proceedings 41, p.127–28, NAI.

Indian Medical Gazette, vol. 56, 1921.

Israili, A. H. "Education of Unani Medicine during Mughal Period." *Studies in History of Medicine* IV, no.3 (1980): 177–82.

Jackson, J.A. ed. *Professions and Professionalization.* Cambridge: Cambridge University Press, 1970.

Jaggi, O. P. "Indian Systems of Medicine during British Supremacy in India," Studies in History of Medicine 1, no. 4 (June 1977): 320–347.

——."Indigenous Medicine during British Supremacy in India." *Studies in History of Medicine* I, no. 4 (1977): 32047.

——."Indigenous System of Medicine during British Supremacy in India." *Studies in History of Medicine* 1, no.4 (Dec.1977): 320–41.

——. "Introduction," Pp. iii–xxii, in *History of Science, Philosophy and Culture in Indian Civilization General,* edited by D. P. Chattopadhyaya. Delhi: Oxford University Press, *Series,* IX, pt I.

——.*Medicine in India: Modern Period.* Delhi: Oxford University Press, 2000.

——.*Medicine in Medieval India.* Delhi: Atma Ram, 1977.

Jalil, A. "The Evolution of Development of Greco-Arab Medical Education." *Studies in History of Medicine* ii, no. 3 (1978): 190–197.

Jee, B. S. H. H. Sir. *A Short History of Aryan Medical Science.* London: MacMillan & Company, 1896.

Jeffery, R. *The Politics of Health in India.* Berkeley: University Press, 1988.

——."Recognizing India's Doctors: The Institutionalization of Medical Dependency (1918–39)." *Modern Asian Studies* 13, no.2 (1979): 301–326.

Johnson, T .J. *Professions and Power.* London: Macmillan, 1972.

Johnston, E. H. *Early Samkhya.* Delhi: Motilal Banarsidass, 1974.

Jolly, J. *Indian Medicine,* trans. C. G. Kashikar, 2nd rev. ed. New Delhi: Munshiram Manoharlal, 1977.

Jones, W. H. S. *Philosophy and Medicine in Ancient Greece.* Baltimore: The Johns Hopkins University Press, 1946.

Jones, W. "Discourse on the Institution of a Society." *Asiatic Researches* xi (1788).

Joshi, L. *Studies in the Buddhistic Culture of India.* Delhi: Motiial Banarsidass, 1964.

Keay, F.E. *Ancient Indian Education,* 122, cited by Edwardes and Garrett, *Mughal Rule in India* (Delhi: S. Chand and Company, 1956), 226–227.

Kelleher, D. and G. Williams (eds.), *Challenging Medicine.* Routledge: London and New York, 1994.

Kelleher, D., J. Gabe and G. Williams, "Understanding Medical Dominnce in the Modem World." Pp. xi–xxix in *Challenging Medicine,* 1994.

Kenoyer, J. M. *Ancient Cities of the Indus Valley Civilization.* Karachi: Oxford University Press, 1998.

Keswani, N. H. *Medical Education in India since Ancient Times* (paper presented at the International Symposium) California, 1968.

Khan, I. A. Khan. "The Middle Classes in the Mughal Empire." *Social Scientist* 5, no. 1, (1977): 2849.

Khan, I. G. "Scientific Concepts in Abul Fazl's Ain-I Akbari." Pp.121–28 in Akbar and his India, edited by Irfan Habib. Delhi: Oxford University Press, 1997.

Khory, R. N. and N. N. Katrak. *The Bombay Materia Medico and Their Therapeutics.* Bombay: Times of India Press, 1903.

King, L. S. *The Medical World of the Eighteenth Century.* New York: Robert Krieger, 1958.

Kingsley, J. D. *Representative Bureaucracy: An Interpretation of the British Civil Service.* Ohio: Yellow Springs, 1944.

Kleinman, A. *Writing at the Margin: Discourse between Anthropology and Medicine.* Berkeley: University of California Press, 1995.

Kopf, D. *British Orientalism and Bengal Renaissance: The Dynamics of Indian Modernization,* 1773–1835. Berkeley: University of California Press, 1969.

Kuhn, T. S. *Structure of Scientific Revolutions.* 1970.

Kulke, H. and D. Rothermund. *A History of India.* London: Routledge, 1990.

Kumar, D. ed. *Science and Empire: Essays in the Indian Context (1700–1947). Delhi:* Anamika, 1991.

Kutumbiah, P. *Ancient Indian Medicine.* Madras: V. Abdullah, 1962.

Leitner, G. *History of Indigenous Education in the Punjab since Annexation and in 1882.* Calcutta: Superintendent of Government Printing, 1882.

Leslie, C. ed. *Asian Medical Systems: A Comparative Study.* Berkeley: University of California Press, 1976.

——. "Modern India's Ancient Medicine." *Transaction* (June 1969): 46–55.

Liebeskind, C. "Arguing Science: Unani *tibb,* Hakims and Biomedicine in India, 1900–50." Pp.58–75 in *Plural Medicine, Tradition,* edited by Waltraud Ernst.

Lupton, D. *Medicine as Culture: Illness, Disease and the Body in Western Societies.* Sage: London, 1994.

Mahabharata. chapters 66 and 84.

Major, R. *H. A History of Medicine.* Oxford: Blackwell, 1954.

Majumdar, R. C. "Medicine." Pp. 213–68 in *A Concise History of Science,* edited by D. M. Bose. New Delhi: Indian National Science Academy, 1971.

Malinowski, B. *A Scientific Theory of Culture and Other Essays.* New York: Oxford University Press, 1960.

Manucci, N. *Storio Do Mogor or Mughal India, 1653–1708,* trans. W. Irvine, II (London, 1907), 176,179, and 214–227.

Marti-Ibanez, F. ed. *Henry Sigerist On the History of Medicine.* New York: MD Publications, Inc., 1960.

McCully, B.T. *English Education and The Origins of Indian Nationalism.* Gloucester: Peter Smith, 1966.

McGuire, J. *The Making of a Colonial Mind: A Quantitative Study of the Bhadralok in Calcutta, 1857–1885.* Canberra: Australian National University, 1983.

Medical Proceedings, no.232 (1835), NAI.

Mehta, H. R. *A History of the Growth and Development of Western Education in Punjab: 1846–1886* (Punjab Government Records), 13–14.

Merson, M.H., R. E. Black, and A. J. Mills. eds., *International Public Health: Diseases. Programs, and Policies,* Maryland: Aspen Publishers, 2001.

Metcalf, B.D. "Nationalist Muslims in British India: The Case of Hakim Ajmal Khan." *Modern Asian Studies* 19, no. 1 (1985): 128.

Meulenbeld, G. J. "Reflections on the Basic Concepts of Indian Pharmacology," Pp. 1–17 in *Studies on Indian Medical History,* edited by G. Jan Meulenbeld and Dominik Wu-jastyk. Groningen: Egbert Forsten, 1987.

Meulenbeld, G.J. and Wujastyk, D. eds. *Studies on Indian Medical History.* Groningen: Egbert Forsten, 1987.

Mirza, H. D. K. *Outlines of Parsi History.* Bombay: Dastur Kayoji Mirza, 1974.

Mishra, S. K. "Tradition of Ayurveda: Evolution and Growth." Pp. 30–915 in *A Concise History of Science in India,* edited by D. M. Bose. New Delhi: Indian National Science Academy, 1971.

Mukherjee, T. and I. Habib. "Akbar and the Temples of Mathura and its Environs." *Proceedings of the Indian History Congress. 48th Session,* Goa, 1987: 234–50.

Mukhopadhyaya, *G. History of Indian Medicine,* vol. II. Calcutta: University of Calcutta, 1926.

Murthy, K. R. S. "Salyatantra (Surgery)." Pp. 325–35 in *A Concise History,* edited by D. M. Bose, *A Concise History of Science in India.* New Delhi: Indian National Science Academy, 1971.

Muthu, D. Chowry. *The Antiquity of Hindu Medicine and Civilisation.* New York: Paul Hoeber, 1931.

Nagel, Ernst. *Teleology Revisited and Other Essays in the Philosophy and History of Science.* New York: Columbia University Press, 1974.

Needham, Joseph, ed., *Science and Civilization in China.* Cambridge: Cambridge University Press, 1954–95.

——.*The Grand Titration: Science and Society in East and West.* London: Allen and Unwin, 1966 and 1969.

Ninivaggi, F. J. *An Elementary Textbook of Ayurveda.* Madison: Psychosocial Press, 2001.

Nutton, V. "Healers in the Medical Market Place: Towards a Social History of Greco-Roman Medicine." Pp. 15–58 in *Medicine in Society: Historical Essays,* edited by A. Wear. Cambridge: Cambridge University Press, 1992.

Official Correspondence, Officiating Deputy Secretary, Government of India, to Chief Commissioner Delhi, Home, B File no.70, 1920, NAI.

O'Flaherty, W.D. ed., *Karma and Rebirth in the Indian Classical Tradition,* Berkeley: University of California Press, 1980.

Osier, W. *The Growth of Truth As Illustrated In the Discovery of the Circulation of the Blood. Selected Writings of Sir William Osier.* Oxford, 1906.

Pandey, B. N. *The Break-up of British India.* London: Macmillan, 1969.

Pannikar, K.N. *Culture. Ideology, Hegemony: Intellectuals and Social Consciousness in Colonial India.* London: Anthem Press, 1995.

Park, K. "Medicine and Society in Medieval Europe: 500–1500." Pp. 59–90 in *Medicine in Society,* edited by A. Wear! Cambridge: Cambridge University Press, 1992.

Parke, Davis and Company, *Great Moments in Medicine-A History of Medicine in Pictures,* Stories by George A. Bender, paintings by Robert A. Thom. Detroit: Northwood Institute Press, 1966.

Patel, B. B. *Parsi.* Bombay: Prakash, vols. I–IV.

Popper, K. *Conjectures and Refutations.* New York: Basic Books, 1963.

Porter, R. and W. F. Bynum. "The Art and Science of Medicine," Pp. 3–11 in *Companion Encyclopedia of the History of Medicine,* edited by Roy Porter and W.F. Bynum. London: Routledge, 1993, vol. I.

Porter, R. *The Greatest Benefit of Mankind: A Medical History of Humanity from Antiquity to the Present.* London: Harper Collins, 1997.

Possehl, G.L. ed. *Ancient Cities of the Indus.* North Carolina: Carolina Academic Press, 1979.

Possehl, G.L. *Indus Age: The Beginnings.* Philadelphia: University of Pennsylvania Press, 1999.

Prakash, G. *Another Reason: Science and the Imagination of Modern India.* Princeton: Princeton University Press, 1999.

Proceedings of the Government of India, Home Department, September–October, 1837.

Qureshi, I. H., *History of the Muslim community in the Indian Subcontinent,* ch. I, 1962, "cited by Percival Spear, *A History of India* (Middlesex: Penguin Books, 1985), vol. 2, 221.

Radhakrishnan, S. *Indian Philosophy.* New York: MacMillan Company, 1962.

Radhakrishnan, S. *Indian Philosophy,* 1923,1, 271–76, quoted in D. P. Chattopadhyaya, *Lokayata: A Study in Ancient Indian Materialism.Nevt* Delhi: People's Publishing House, 1959.

Rahman, A. *The Cultural and Philosophical Roots of Scientific Traditions.* Delhi: National Institute of Science, Technology and Development Studies, 1983.

Rahman, A. "Science and Technology in Medieval India: Introduction to a Bibliography of Source Material in Sanskrit, Arabic and Persian." *Cressida Transactions* 1, no.1 (1981): 187–98.

Raj, K.C.K.E. *A Note on Chopra Committee's Report on Indigenous Medicine,* vol. 1, Directorate General of Health Services, 1949.

Raj, K.N. "Politics and Economics of Intermediate Regimes." *Economic and Political Weekly* viii, no.27 (7 July 1973): 1191.

Report of Government of India Committee on Indigenous Systems of Medicine (Chopra Committee), File 1105/1949, Medical (B) Department, Uttar Pradesh State Archives (UPSA).

Report of the All India Ayurvedic Conference. Seventh Session, Madras, 1915.

Report of the Health Survey and Development Committee, vol. II– IV (Delhi, 1946).

Report of the Health Survey and Planning Committee, vol. I, Delhi, 1962.

Resolution no. 11, Adopted by the Central Provincial Health Ministers' Conference, New Delhi, 1946.

Richards, John F. *The New Cambridge History of India: The Mughal Empire.* Cambridge: Cambridge University Press, 1993.

Richardson, R. *Death, Dissection and the Destitute,* London: Penguin, 1988.

Risse, G.B. "Medicine in the Age of Enlightenment." Pp. 149–95 in *Medicine in Society,* edited by A. Cambridge: Cambridge University Press, 1992.

Robinson, F. *Separatism among Indian Muslims: The Politics of the United Provinces Muslims, 1860–1923.* Cambridge: Cambridge University Press, 1974.

Saiyid, A. ed., *Tuzuk-e-Jahangiri, Ghazipur and Aligar (1863–64).*

Saks, M. "Removing the Blinkers? A Critique of Recent Contributions to the Sociology of Professions." *Sociological Review,* 31, no. 1 (1983): 1–21.

Sanskrit College, General Records and Correspondence, 1827–55.

Sarkar, J. N. ed., *Later Mughals,* 311, cited by S.M. Edwards and H.L.O. Garrett. *Mughal Rule in India.*

Scheper-Huges, N. and M.M. Lock, "The Mindful Body: A Proleomenon to future work in Medical Anthropology," *Medical Anthropology Quarterly,* 1, (1987): 6–41.

Seal, A. *The Emergence of Indian Nationalism.* Cambridge: Cambridge University Press, 1968.

Sen, S.N. "A Survey of Source Materials." in *A Concise History of Science in India,* edited by D. M. Bose. New Delhi: Indian National Science Academy, 1971.

Siddiqui, M.Z. "The Unani-Tibb (Greek Medicine) in India." in *A Concise History of Science in India* edited by D.M.Bose. New Delhi: Indian National Science Academy, 1971.

Siddiqui, T. "Unani Medicine in India." *Indian Journal of History of Science* 16, no. 1 (May 1981): 22–5.

——. "Unani Medicine in India during the Delhi Sultanate." *Studies in History of Medicine* II, no.3 (1978): 183–89.

Sigerist, H. *A History of Medicine,* vol. II. New York: Oxford University Press, 1961.

Sinh Jee, B. (Thakore Saheb of Golconda). *A Short History of Aryan Medical Science.* London: MacMillan and Company, 1896.

Sobel, D. *Galileo's Daughter.* New York: Walker and Company, 1999.

——. *Letters to Father (Suor Maria Celeste) to Galileo (1623–1633),* translated and annotated by Dava Sobel. New York: Walker and Co., 2001.

Spear, P. *A History of India,* vol. 2. Middlesex: Penguin Books, 1978,1985.

Steinthal, B. J. "The Ayurvedic Revivalist Movement in Early Twentieth-Century British India." (B.A. thesis, Harvard University, 1984).

Thakur, V. K. *Urbanisation in Ancient India.* Delhi: Abhinav Publications, 1981.

——.*Towns in Pre-Modern India.* New Delhi: Janaki Prakashan, 1994.

Thapar, R. "Imagined Religious Communities? Ancient History and the Modern Search for a Hindu Identity," in *History and Beyond,* edited by Romila Thapar. New Delhi: Oxford University Press, 2000.

The Asiatic Society (1784–1984), Bicentenary Report (Calcutta, 1985).

Thorner, D. *The Shaping of Modem India.* New Delhi: R. N. Sachdev, 1980.

Udupa, K. N. "The Health System in India." in *Health by The People,* edited by K.W. Newell. Geneva: WHO, 1975.

Underwood, E. A., ed. vol. 2. London: Oxford University Press, 1953.

Venkataraman, C. R. "A History of Medicine in India (1664–1945)." *Indian Journal of History of Medicine* 19, no. 1, (1974): 5–14.

Verna, R. L. and N. H. Keswani. "Unani Medicine in Medieval India: Its Teachers and Texts" in *The Science of Medicine and Physiological Concepts in Ancient and Medieval India,* edited by N. H. Keswani. New Delhi: S. K. Manchanda, 1974: 127–42.

Verma, R. L. Verna and N. H. Keswani. "Women in the Arabic Medicine." *Studies in the History of Medicine* (Dec.1977): 271–84.

Wear, A., ed. *Medicine in Society: Historical Essays.* Cambridge: Cambridge University Press, 1992.

Weiss, M. G. "Caraka Samhita on the Doctrines of Karma," Pp.90–115 in *Karma and Rebirth in the Indian Classical Tradition,* edited by W. D. O'Flaherty. Berkeley: University of California Press, 1980.

Winther, P.C. *Anglo-European Science and the Rhetoric of Empire: Malaria, Opium, and British Rule in India, 1756–1895.* New York: Lexington Books, 2003.

Weiss, M., A. Cohen, and L. Eisenberg. "Mental Health," Pp.331–377 in *International Public Health: Diseases, Programs, and Policies,* edited by Michael H. Merson, Robert E. Black, and Anne J. Mills. Maryland: Aspen Publishers, 2001.

Wise, T. *Commentary on the Hindu System of Medicine.* London: Trubner, 1860.

Wolf, A. *A History of Science, Technology and Philosophy in Sixteenth and Seventeenth Centuries,* vol. II. Gloucester: Peter Smith, 1968.

Zachariah, B. "Uses of Scientific Argument: The Case of' Development in India', c 1930–1950." *Economic and Political Weekly* (Sept. 29, 2001): 3689–702.

Zahuri, A.W. "Development of Greco-Arab Literature in India." *Studies in History, of Medicine* iii, no 2 (1979): 125–45.

Zysk, K. *Religious Healing in the Vedas, Transactions of the American Philosophical Society,* vol. 75 (7). Philadelphia: The American Philosophical Society, 1985.

——."Mantra in Ayurvcda: A Study of the Use of Magico-Religious Speech in Ancient India," in *Understanding Mantra,* edited by Harvey Alper. New York: SUNY Press, 1985.

Index

About the Author

Poonam Bala has taught in various universities in Canada, USA, and India, including her teaching tenure at Case Western Reserve University in Cleveland, Ohio, and most recently, as a Reader (Associate Professor) at the Delhi School of Economics, University of Delhi. As a Course Director in Sociology of Health and Health Care at York University, Canada, a Wellcome Fellow at the Institute of History of Medicine in London, and an Honorary Fellow at the Institute of Advanced Studies in the Humanities at the University of Edinburgh, Bala has been one of the Consultants to a discussion forum on the globalization of *Ayurveda,* at the Faculty of Divinity, University of Cambridge, UK. Her earlier work, *Imperialism and Medicine in Bengal: A Socio-Historical Perspective* is, by far, one of the few region-specific writings on history of medicine in the non-Western world in a colonial setting. Bala has been on the Advisory Board of Ancient Science of Life (a journal of the International Institute of *Ayurveda),* and invited on the Board of Scientific Sessions at the history of science conferences in Mexico and Beijing. She has studied at the University of Delhi, Jawaharlal Nehru University (New Delhi), and at the University of Edinburgh, (UK), where she obtained her doctoral degree in Sociology.

www.ingramcontent.com/pod-product-compliance
Lightning Source LLC
LaVergne TN
LVHW101448200926
848483LV00001B/94
9780739113226